BEDTIME STORIES
FOR ADULTS & FOR KIDS

More than 50 stories to listen in family.

Say goodbye to insomnia, anxiety and panic
attacks. Whit advanced meditation and
hypnosis techniques.

Katherine Bennett

TABLE OF CONTENTS

BEDTIME STORIES FOR ADULTS

2

TABLE OF CONTENTS

BEDTIME STORIES FOR KIDS

BEDTIME STORIES
FOR ADULTS

27 Stories

With deep Hypnosis for stress, panic
attacks, anxiety relief, meditation

And relaxed sleep

Katherine Bennet

Introduction

First, let's talk about why do bedtime stories matter?

Well, do you remember going to bed as a child, hearing those wonderful stories your mom or dad, or even your guardian, tell you?

Those stories were a focal point of many children's lives. And, for most of us, remembering the fond memories that came with hearing those tales was something that helped many of us go to sleep within a reasonable time period, and have pleasant dreams.

Mindfulness, relaxation, and hypnotizing the body into a pleasant sleep is a key part of all this. The stories that you heard were whimsical tales, and while they might have seemed like much as a child, when looking back on this as an adult, it played a major role in our lives.

Bedtime stories were fun to hear. Sometimes, your parent would do voices. Other times, they'd just read the books quietly, and you'd pay attention each time. Sometimes they'd be tales you've heard plenty of times, other times they were tales they fabricated on a whim.

Regardless of what type of tales you heard, bedtime stories are wonderful for falling asleep. Most of them have soft, pleasant words that people love to hear.

Do you remember some of your former bedtime stories?

If you do, do you remember how they made you feel? The words you heard. The imagery you'd remember.

All of this plays a key role in why bedtime stories for adults are so important, and why, with each story you hear, you feel relaxed, at ease, and of course, able to sleep.

Each story will have fun, whimsical ideas, or imagery of different scenarios that you've been through before. The fun and excitement of going on a trip, the quests that you have, and even, a sleep fairy that will help you sleep. With every single story, you'll be spirited away on a wonderful adventure, one that's fun for you, and a good trip for everyone in the story.

If you have trouble falling asleep, just imagine yourself in the different scenarios each of these wonderful characters go through. As you get spirited away in this adventure, you'll notice that, with each time, and each place, it'll change for you. There are many different aspects to consider with each story, and many adventures to be had.

Also, don't think you'll hear the same story twice. While it might be the same words, there might be new adventures to be had, and new ideas that come forth.

Listening to bedtime stories will help foster your creative juices, help you improve you with ideas for the future, and also reduce stress. By listening to these ten wonderful stories, you'll be able to fall asleep soundly, and you'll be amazed at how refreshed you feel whenever you wake up.

Bedtime stories for adults also help with taking your attention off the troubles of life. If you're an adult, chances are you have some kind of stress. Whether it be work, bills, or even your family, that stress adds up, and it can make it hard for you to fall asleep. Many adults suffer from insomnia or can only sleep for a certain period of hours. That combined with the incredibly long work weeks, and also with the early morning shifts, it's not easy out there. But, with these bedtime stories, you'll relax your mind, you'll take your attention off the troubles you have, and promote relaxation, and of course sleep with each word you hear.

Many adults benefit from these types of stories. Some of us might wonder why, but if you take a moment to think about it, when was the last time you weren't focused on the stresses at hand, but instead on a relaxing, fun bedtime story that will help with sleep. If you can't remember, then you need these bedtime stories for adults.

With each story, each word uttered, each sound you hear, I hope they will lull you to sleep. It helps as well with shutting off your brain, helping you get focused on the different words you hear, and instead of feeling stressed and depressed, you'll get your mind off the troubles you have, and instead, feel brighter than ever.

With each of these stories, as you hear them when you sleep, you'll notice when you wake up you feel refreshed. That's because, with each sound, you'll hear words as well that are relaxing, soothing, and will help with sleep. Instead of stories that will keep you on your feet and alert, these small, short stories are simple, and yet very effective. If you have trouble relaxing, turning your mind off, and lulling the body to sleep, then this is for you. With each passing story, you'll feel your attention slowly slip away. Each sound you hear pulling you into a far-off land, into a realm of sleep that makes you feel happy, and at ease.

So, sit back, get comfortable, and listen to these relaxing bedtime stories. And with every one of these, you'll feel yourself whisked away into the tales they tell, and hopefully, you'll have pleasant dreams and a wonderful sleep as you continue to hear each story, and the creative, relaxing, and inspiring tales each one of them has to offer.

CHAPTER 1

A Journey Through Space and Time

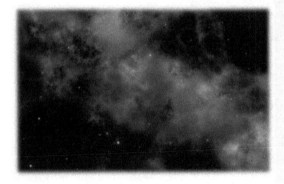

Before we begin this journey downwards into the deepest realms of our sub-conscious, let us take a minute to physically and mentally and spiritually acclimate ourselves into being with awareness of our inner sanctum, our internal workings. We will begin by going to a place of comfort, ideally a bed, or a very comfortable reclining chair, and we will relax our bodies to the furthest extent possible. Now, close your eyes, staying firmly on your back, with your arms relaxed at your sides and your legs rested downwards. Take one deep breath in, through your nostrils, counting slowly to four, and one deep breath out, through your nostrils again, counting slowly to four. Breathe in the breath of the spirit and breathe out the stress of the day. Now is the time to rest. Become aware of nothing but the air flowing through your nostrils, envision a steady flowing stream, smooth inhalations and exhalations, your body become weightier and more relaxed with each passing cycle of breath. Allow your thoughts to become completely still, as you focus on your core, your solar plexus, allowing your thoughts to flow outwards past your vision until they escape your being, while only holding and retaining the pure awareness of spirit, the holy serenity of the mind and body. Breathe in, one, two, three, four, then breathe out, one, two, three, four, each breath becoming slower. One... two... three... four... One... two... three... four... One... two... three... four... One... two... three... four... One... two... three... four... One... two... three... four... Continue this pattern of breath, expanding, and sink down deeper into yourself, becoming a voyeur of your own still, relaxed body, lost in time. Become lost in this experience as you journey further into the trance and prepare for the road we are about to embark upon. Draw further and further away from your still, lying body, and into the realm of imagination, where images grow, the land of dreams that you are about to become one with. Erase your mind of all that is within it currently and prepare the landscape for a new and fresh experience, in the farther reaches of reality. One... two... three... four... inhale... One... two... three... four... exhale... One... two... three... four... inhale... One... two... three... four... exhale... Now, with your mind, body, and spirit rested totally, entranced, and fertile, let us begin.

You are the sun. The galaxy is orbiting around you. You watch as they rotate and spin, and travel in shifting circles around where you stand, intersecting each other by what seems like fractions of an inch, an intricate dance around you. You hold out your hand, and hold it over a big, blue planet that echoes a warm, loving moisture. Tiny pieces of rock hover around it. The orb tingles your hands, and you feel a dearth of electricity course from it and into you and back into it. You are totally electric. You begin to move, floating, walking, out past the galaxy, and you realize that these galaxies are mirror images of each other, repeated over and over, tiny fractals, as far as you can see. You dance from one

11

galaxy to the next, and with each transition you feel a new magnetic pull dancing around you, tiny energies, barely affecting you as you traverse this plane. This miniature, ornate landscape of suns, and moons, and stars, all dancing around each other, these quaint little machines, existing like a trillion little raindrops trickling down through eternity. Beyond you, even beyond all these galaxies, is the universe, what feels to be several lengths of the arm away from you are giant globes of energy, planets that dwarf the sun. You hover around them, and, as you do, you grow to their size, and the previous galaxies you had been born from shrink down to a level at which they are no longer visible. You are flying through space at an imperceptible rate, getting bigger, and bigger, and you know that no matter how large you grow, how exponential the growth is from the size you are now, you will still be nothing to existence but an imperceptible dot, the cage of reality so infinitely large that its barriers cannot be touched by a lifetime of growing at the fastest rate imaginable. You take control of your situation and start flying, like a rocket, hovering past increasingly large galaxies that begin to whiz by you in a great blur. Whereas they used to be identical but perceptible as individual units, now, at this speed, they really become one, and all there is can be summed up as one vibrating, holographic image, akin to frames on a reel of film, projected by at hundreds per second. You begin to wonder if you are still, the universe whizzing by you, or if you really are moving, as you feel that you are, as you told yourself to. Space is illusory. You are stagnant, and floating, and infinite, but always moving, and growing, becoming more. You come upon a gigantic star, many, many times larger than you, and its heat glows gold in a way that doesn't affect your physiology, but only your soul. You are aware that your temperature is at a homeostatic point, independent of anything around you. You are the warmth of your soul, and these are mere physical bodies. The golden glow, however, itself, is on your level. This is affecting you. The golden glow inspires you take it with you. You absorb the golden light of this sun and grow to dwarf the sun, with a glow that dwarfs its own origin. You are now the golden light spreading through the cosmos, unconsciously, merely an experience perpetuating

12

through infinity at a rate that increases in relation to its own size; always growing, faster and faster, spreading, farther and farther, bigger and farther tenfold with each step. There are many black holes, bigger and smaller, and tiny pieces of you are sucked in, and spat out, all across the infinite cosmos. Each piece that is torn asunder is still communicating back to the whole, and with each new individual journey of the part is that much more growth given back to the entire unit. New clouds of gold are spreading, but they are all of a whole, all the same, all right there with you. They grow, and they meet, then they separate and spread, and all the while it is still smaller than a pinprick on the fabric of reality as a whole. This could continue for several infinities and still not make a dent. But it is so large, and so powerful; it is beyond the scope of man, to even perceive such a thing. This is every lifetime of every human that has ever existed, to the power of itself, squared, cubed, to the power of a variable that increases with each step. You have made yourself the source of infinite life in the universe, in the image of whatever came before you, the thing that you have become. It is unknowing, because to know itself would be a waste of time, as it is what it is, and growing, and eternal, and, more than eternal, infinite, to infinite degrees. Rolling past faster than the speed of light, but from a vantage point of such greatness it appears to be a drop of water slowing making its way down a sheet of glass, like a raindrop splattered on a car window. The light reflected off this stream of water houses within it mirror infinites that exist fractured within this one. Many lifetimes housed inside each other, like the tip of a pyramid bleeding down forever with no tangible base, only ethereal and infinite growth. As we fly through space, we become larger and larger, and the distance between our molecules grows exponentially, making it so that at one moment in our lives we may be a trillion times bigger than we were at a moment previous, yet this growth would be imperceptible to the senses because all the senses, as well, are growing with it. Likewise, you begin to wonder how much you have actually grown on your journey through space, in dreams, if it is even quantifiable how much larger you are now than when you started. The swirling, dancing lights around you, that shift around each

13

other as you change your perspective to almost become an infinite, solid wall, made up of tiny dots yet so thoroughly blended and so indistinguishable in their tiny distance apart that it may as well be one singular, shining force, they are all that is. As you have strived for the spread the golden light, the golden light has manifested across the entire solar system as it can be known to you, and while it is still spreading, and will spread forever, you have made a home of it, here, now, and you vibrate in ecstasy, a light within light, indefinable, save for the golden glow that is. You stop, for once, you rest, and you are nothing but the golden light. Forever, all that is, is here, now, completely still, yet growing, imperceptibly, infinitely, flying through space at the speed of light, stagnant, unchanging, for eternity and eternity after that, as you sleep.

CHAPTER 2

Priorities

J ack was a 65-year-old man who was rather proud of the life that he had built for his family. He had worked hard since his teenage years and done everything he could over the past five decades to give his family the life that he felt they deserved. He spent long hours working as a laborer, pulling in as many extra shifts as he could so that he could provide for his family. Thanks to his hard work, his wife was able to stay home and raise their three children in a beautiful home that he had purchased for them. He filled the home full of furniture, food, and various treasures based on whatever his family desired to have. When his family wanted to go on vacation, he would work overtime to afford the added expense and would always plan dreamy vacations that brought his family great joy. They would visit places like Disney Land, Martha's Vineyard, and even Arizona to see the desert. His family traveled to many different places enjoying all of the different views and creating many different memories.

Although he seemed to be around fairly frequently, Jack never felt as though he was able to truly relax and enjoy his time with his family. He had grown so used to working hard that he always had to be doing something: fixing something, building something, cleaning something, or moving something around. No matter what day it was or how much work he had already done, Jack would always do more work than what was reasonable because he simply felt uncomfortable just sitting around and enjoying the presence of his family. To Jack, nothing felt more satisfying than retiring after a hard day of working and feeling the comfort of his pillow rising to meet him.

One day, when he turned 66, Jack found that he was not feeling as good as he used to. For a while, he chalked it up to being older and dealing with regular pains of old age. After a few months, however, Jack could no longer deny that he was experiencing some fairly serious symptoms. His symptoms had grown so strong that he could no longer do the labor work that he once had, so he quit his job and retired to please his family. If it were up to him, Jack would have found a way to keep working despite his setbacks with his health. Still, he listened and retired, as he knew he probably should.

Shortly into his retirement, even simple things became challenging for Jack. He could no longer work like he used to, and eventually, even smaller tasks like climbing the stairs or going for a walk to the mailbox became more of a challenge for him. Finally, with his family's insistence, Jack went to visit a doctor to see why he might be experiencing such hardship with his health. It was from that appointment that Jack went on to learn that he was terminally ill with cancer and that he had waited too long to be checked so he was beyond the point of being able to be cured.

Jack and his family were shocked by this news as they realized that the once vital and virile man was quickly falling apart before their very eyes. Within weeks, Jack could no longer climb the stairs at all, and sometimes he even had troubles holding his coffee mug or pouring himself a glass of water. His wife, Susan, had to do everything for him. Being unable to do anything for himself made Jack angry and embarrassed, as he had always been a very proud and self-sufficient man. He spent the past five decades taking care of this woman; he did not feel as though he needed his wife to be taking care of him, now.

As time went on, Jack's anger turned into sadness. His family would all visit him in his home and bring their young children around, and everyone would play and get along like they always had. This time, though, Jack was forced to sit there and observe and partake in the conversation as he could no longer get up and find some work to do to keep himself busy. It was during these visits that Jack grew to

16

understand just how much he had missed by being so deeply devoted to his work ethic and not spending enough time paying attention to his family. He realized that he had missed countless birthdays, holidays, anniversaries, and even just simple day-to-day memories because he was so absorbed in his need to work that he never truly sat down to enjoy his family until it was almost too late.

At first, Jack was angry with himself for not having spent more time with his family. He could not understand how foolish he had been by working so intensely and missing out on the majority of his children's and grandchildren's lives. Then, he became angry that he felt he had no choice but to work that hard to be able to give them the life that he wanted them all to enjoy. Eventually, Jack found himself thanking his own life for giving him enough time to see what he had missed and for giving him the opportunity to make up for it now before it was too late.

One day, when he was talking to his son, Jack decided to offer him some advice about his work ethic. Jack said, "Son, when I was your age my priorities were all wrong. I thought I had to work the hardest, be the best, and make the most money to make my family happy. Your mother told me she wanted me around more and wished I was there for the kids more, and I justified my actions by saying that I was there financially to support them. But that's not enough, son. In life, simply giving someone our money and hard work is not enough. If you truly want to be happy and live your best life, you take some time every single day to sit with those kids of yours and enjoy them. Never work so hard that you miss birthdays, anniversaries, or even just those special suppers each night. Be there for as many moments as you can, son, because believe me, one day they will have all slipped by. I realize now my priorities were wrong, and I taught you wrong. The true priority you need to have in life is to be able to provide for your family, but not just with finances. Prioritize the opportunity to provide them with your time, your attention, and your love. Believe me, son. It will make a world of difference."

Jack's son never forgot this story and went on to live by these words even long after Jack had passed. In fact, Jack's son went on to teach his

17

own children about the value of these priorities, and they went on to teach their children! So, thanks to Jack and his hard work, his entire family was able to enjoy more quality time together for generations to come because he took the time to realize that prioritizing finances was not the only important thing in life. Time, attention, and love also mattered when it comes to providing for your family and truly taking care of them, and yourself.

CHAPTER 3

Daddy and Daughter's Fishing Trip

I will tell you a story of a young girl who keeps wanting to spend some time with her dad, but her dad is always busy, her dad is always working or wanting to relax and have time for himself.

Every day the girl asks;

"Will you spend time with me today?"

And every day he is always too busy. Eventually just as she is giving up hope and yet still keeps trying, he responds by saying he wants to take her fishing, he wants to teach her how to fish. The girl didn't really have an interest in fishing, but was interested in spending time with her father, so the two of them, the next morning, woke up, packed for the fishing trip and set off to a nearby lake. As they arrived at the lake, so the girl looked around. She enjoyed the smell of that fresh air, the breeze on her face, there were a few clouds in the sky. She could see trees around the edge of the lake and lush grass. No-one else seemed to be around. Her father said took her down to a boat.

He carried a lot of the fishing gear as she carried a little. They got on the boat. The father started to row out into the middle of the lake and then the daughter asked if she could have a go at rowing and so she rowed that boat towards the middle of the lake. At first, she struggled to get the coordination between the left and the right oar and they kept going around in circles and then weaving the other way and then the other way and sometimes the oar wouldn't go into the water right and it would splash water up into her father's face and he was laughing with her and she was laughing at him.

And they rowed out into the middle of the lake, pulled the oars onto the boat and just allowed the boat to bob up and down in the middle of the lake. The father then baited the fishing hook and demonstrated how to get that hook as far away from the boat as possible into the water. And he whipped that rod as the reel un-spun and the hook shot off and plopped into the water. She then got her smaller fishing rod and facing the opposite side of the boat, she copied her dad and whipped the rod and almost straightaway got it right by copying him. And the hook plopped into the water. And he said

"You just have to sit and wait, just sit silently and patiently and feel the rod, feel any subtle movement, sensations. What you are looking for is a sign that a fish has bitten on the bait and a slight tug on that hook and that slight tug with translate into a slight movement at the tip of the rod which will be felt at the handle and you just have to be able to sit and wait and focus on the feelings, focus on the sensations. It's about becoming in tune with those feelings and sensations, learning to notice the most subtle response and to be able to begin to learn the difference between a lifeless piece of weed catching on that hook and a fish and you can begin to learn the different way both feel, the different way different things feel, through your fingertips, through the palms of your hands holding onto that rod, so that you will know when to reel that fish in. And when reeling a fish in, it is about sensitivity, reel too fast and you will lose the fish, reel too slow and you will lose the fish, so you have to reel at just the right speed, which requires sensitivity to know when to reel faster or slower and when to pause reeling in or reeling out and it is almost like falling into a dance with the fish on the end of that line. And so, it is with many other things in life, all you have to do is learn to transfer skills from one area to another. There are people you need to deal with in life, like fish and situations you need to deal with like this and so fishing will teach more about life than just how to fish."

The girl had a sense that she kind of understood, but she didn't know how you transfer skills from one part of life to another, but she trusted that somehow it must happen, and she was enjoying her fishing trip with her father. It was these kinds of experiences that she wanted, something where she learned from the wisdom of her dad. After a few hours of fishing on that lake, her father had caught a few fish and yet nothing had bitten her line. And she was wondering whether she was doing something wrong. So, the father taught her a trick, a way of wiggling the rod, of pulling the line in and out a little bit to create movement at the hook, which creates curiosity and intrigue. She did this and suddenly she got a bite and excitedly she started reeling in this fish, following her father's instructions, not too fast, not too slow, sometimes letting the line go, sometimes pulling the line in, pulling on the rod and loosening the rod and eventually she got the fish to the boat. She had a photo taken with that fish before she unhooked it and threw it back and then she decided it was starting to get a bit late and she was starting to get hungry. It was just after lunch time and she had been there for hours, so the father suggested, why don't they row down the river, as he knows this nice place to stop.

The father and his daughter set off across the lake to the river and started rowing down the river. They rowed past people walking on the bank and she loved just sitting back, closing her eyes and feeling the warmth of the sun and the breeze on her face, as they rowed, as she listened to the sound of the oars, as they pushed the water behind them while she would occasionally talk to her father and he would talk back and she had this strong feeling that she was creating something beautiful in her mind which will last with her forever. And as they carried on rowing, they saw dog walkers on the shore, some people just sitting there eating sandwiches, some people waved and said hello, for no reason at all other than that they were passing by and after a little while they arrived at a little pier area, somewhere to dock up the boat and so the father navigated the boat alongside the pier, tied the boat to the side, helped his daughter off and then climbed off the boat himself.

They were at a beautiful country hotel. They walked up to the hotel and were going to the restaurant of this hotel. They sat outside overlooking the river. The father went into the hotel, got some menus and returned, they looked at the menus and decided what they would like to eat. Someone came outside and served them, they ordered a couple of drinks and ordered their food and they sat just peacefully with the mumble of voices in the background, just sat and enjoyed the view, enjoyed gazing over the river, watching others in boats of different kinds occasionally pass by, enjoying some relaxing time with dad and daughter.

Then their food came out, they ate their food and had a little talk with each other about their interests, mainly the dad asking what the daughter liked to do, asking what was going on in her life at the moment. While her mouth was answering her mind was thinking about the fact that he was totally focused on her, he wasn't thinking about work, thinking about other things, thinking about what time he had to go, he appeared totally interested in her and what she had to say and totally in that moment with her and she felt so loved and valued and respected in that moment and knew that her father being like this, was teaching her more than just giving her a nice experience as a dad. Teaching her about the way people interact and communicate meaningfully with each other and after eating, they had another drink and continued sitting there and she realized it was now getting well into the afternoon and the sun was beginning to set. The sky was starting to turn the most beautiful orange.

They left the hotel and went and sat on the pier with their feet dangling over the edge, just continuing talking as the sun started getting lower over the horizon and then before the sun had fully set the dad said it was time to start heading back home. To head down the river, back to that lake and back to the shore before it gets too dark. And as the sun was beginning its journey over the horizon they got back in the boat and the dad rowed the boat back along the river towards the lake and the daughter continued to savor this moment, to savor this day. And then they arrived at the lake, the moon was more visible in the sky now, starting to shine brightly. The sun was almost totally set, it had long gone over the horizon, but there was enough light still to just about make out the shore, so the dad rowed to the shore and he said to his daughter "do you want to know how to start a fire? And do you want an experience

22

of camping, just for a few hours, to really make the end of this day special?" He thought this would round off the day. Obviously when they get home they will go to bed, but for now she could have this experience and he could teach her about camping.

The daughter wanted this experience, so together they gathered up some wood from among the nearby trees, he demonstrated clearing an area to make sure the fire wouldn't set fire to anything it isn't supposed to, he demonstrated stacking the wood and making it so that it would light and then he lit the fire and the daughter got two chairs out of the car, set up those chairs near the fire. The dad got some food out of an ice box and they cooked up that food and enjoyed watching the last of the sunlight, watching how the stars appeared more in the sky twinkling above, the way the moonlight now glistened on the lake and then after a little while the dad said it was time for them to go home, so they put out the fire, packed everything away and made their journey back home. And on the journey home the daughter and the dad continued talking and bonding and the daughter said she wanted to do this kind of thing more often, she didn't want it to be just a one-off.

The dad said he needed to make more effort, he said he could get so wrapped up in work, in what he feels he needs to do, so that he forgets to focus on what he should do and sometimes life can pass you by while you are busy focusing on something else and when there are loved ones involved you don't want that to be the case and he told her the trip had taught him a lot about where his priorities should be and how he should focus his attention. And the daughter closed her eyes and just listened as the car drove along, just listened to the sounds around them, with a smile on her face, reminiscing about the day she has just had and hoping that this is the first of many. On arriving home, she kissed her dad, went up to bed, got into bed and allowed herself to drift into a pleasant dream as she began to drift off comfortably asleep.

CHAPTER 4

Forgiveness

C hloe and Joy had been friends for many years. They grew up in the same town together, with their houses right next door to each other. They met when they were around four years old, when Joy moved in next to Chloe. For years, the two of them would play together, running around the neighborhood playing tag, pretending that sticks were their swords, and playing in Chloe's backyard treehouse. The two were practically inseparable, as they rode the bus to school together, went to the same class, played together after school, and slept over at each other's houses all the time. When they reached high school, they had some classes together and some classes apart, yet they still spent the majority of their time together. They would spend lunch hour together talking about their homework and boys, get ready for school together in the morning, and carpool to school each day. On weekends, they attended their boyfriend's sporting events or the party of the weekend, or they would simply catch a movie together. To put it simply, they did everything together.

When they graduated, Chloe and Joy were excited to attend college together. They had both applied at all of the same colleges and universities and had agreed that they would go to a school together and share an apartment off campus together, as they had dreamed of this their entire lives. In senior year while they were applying to colleges and universities, they also found that a few other things in their lives were changing. Joy had met a boy who she really liked and started dating, and the two started hanging out more frequently. Chloe grew frustrated when Joy was no longer hanging out with her, but Joy knew that Chloe would get over it eventually. Unfortunately, Chloe never did get over it.

24

The argument grew even more complicated when Joy chose to go to the same school as her boyfriend rather than the same school as Chloe, and Chloe could not attend that school, as she had not been accepted.

When they graduated and left for college, Joy, and Chloe were not even talking anymore as Chloe was so hurt by Joy's actions. Joy was sad that Chloe was hurt but was also frustrated that Chloe was not being supportive of Joy's romance and desires to make her own path in life. The two were so frustrated at each other that they hardly talked through freshman and sophomore year. However, in junior year they were both at home at the same time and crossed each other's paths in the driveway. Chloe was mad, but Joy wanted to reconcile. She did her best to explain to Chloe what had happened and that she was sorry, but Chloe was not interested in hearing what Joy had to say. She ignored Joy and walked to her car and took off, and Joy hardly ever saw Chloe after that. From that day forward, the two never connected when they were at home, even if they saw each other outside they would just pretend that the other did not exist.

One day after they had both graduated, Joy's family decided to sell the family home and move away to a new state. Joy no longer returned back to the family home, which meant that she never had the potential of running into Chloe in the driveway anymore. In a way, she was relieved that she would not have to run into that awkward encounter anymore. In another way, Joy was upset that it felt like she would never have the chance to reconcile with her old best friend. She knew that after her family sold and moved away, it was unlikely that she would ever be able to get back in touch with her friend, which meant that the relationship was officially over, for good.

Chloe was also sad when she saw that Joy's family had moved. For her, knowing that Joy would always be there or coming back was comforting, as she knew that there would always be the chance that the two of them would reconcile and save their friendship. After Joy's family had moved, it became apparent that this chapter was officially closed. Chloe was disappointed in herself for not treating Joy better and for being unwilling to see the whole reality, as this led to Joy thinking that Chloe was unwilling to reconcile the relationship.

For years, as the two grew their careers, raised their families, and lived their separate lives, they both experienced intense guilt around the end of their relationship. Both women wished that they had contributed to finding reconciliation more so that they could have lived their lives together. They missed calling each other and sharing moments together and always wished that they could have grown together through these later parts of life. Despite the fact that Joy went on to marry her high school sweetheart whom she went to college with, she always wished that she would have chosen to go to school with Chloe or put more effort into keeping their friendship alive. Chloe always wished that she had not been so stubborn and that she had been willing to see things from Joy's perspective, especially once she realized that Joy and her now husband's relationship was serious. At the time, Chloe thought it would be a short-term fling and felt betrayed by Joy's lack of loyalty, but she no longer saw it this way. Still, it felt like it was too late for them to reconcile, so they both kept their guilt to themselves and refused to do anything about it.

One day, Joy was walking through the grocery store when she saw a familiar face. "Chloe? Is that you?" She asked, walking up to the lady by the fruit. "Joy?" Chloe asked, shocked. "I thought you family left this area?" She asked, looking at Joy. "They did, but Ronald and I moved back recently." Joy smiled. The two talked in the produce section of the grocery store for nearly an hour before swapping numbers and agreeing to meet up with each other. They both apologized for their actions and forgave each other, realizing now that their feud had gone on far too long and that the consequences were far harsher than the action itself. The ladies realized that their friendship was strong and that there was no amount of time or space that could prevent them from being each other's best friends.

Over the next several weeks, they caught each other up on their lives and began hanging out again on a regular basis. They talked as if nothing had changed, and they spent plenty of time together bonding once again. They realized that they had believed forgiveness would be harder than it truly was and that they had both lost a lot of time with each other due to their unwillingness to forgive each other. From that day forward, Chloe and Joy remained best friends. They also learned that if they were ever going through something with a loved one, it was better to find a way to reconcile and to mend the relationship, rather than allowing years of guilt and hurt to pass first.

CHAPTER 5

Micah's Story

There's no sympathy for the person a universe revolves around. It's not the universe's fault. It's not anyone's fault. The problem was, as Micah observed, his universe only got as big as it needed to.

So, he felt like he was the only person in the world going through anything. Even when his parents genuinely believed they understood, they didn't. Their "sympathy" seemed synthetic, and in the end, Micah really wanted empathy. But no one could give him empathy, because only one person could be the center of the universe. And it was him.

One day, late into his junior year of high school, Micah realized why everything was the way it was. Micah was particularly observant, and he could even tell when his world was missing an amplitude of potential detail. He learned that an author couldn't possibly hope to describe everything about a place. Anything an author left out of description had to be assumed or interpreted by a reader. Micah wasn't the reader - he was part of the world. And he was the most important part because things only happened when they related directly or indirectly to himself. That's how stories are.

But it was a long road until Micah solved this mystery.

Micah used his sheltering parents to his advantage even when he was five years old. In the back of his mind, he somehow knew it was all about him. He hadn't learned the word "protagonist" yet, but he'd already embraced that identity.

He figured out that the point of his childhood was to show how insightful he was. Nothing else. Things didn't happen unless they emphasized this fact; his childhood life passed like a montage in a movie.

By the end of it, Micah realized that less interesting things had to exist. Surely the universe let things happen that didn't have purpose. Maybe there were fewer coincidences than one would think, but they couldn't be nonexistent! In his life, they were nonexistent. Every event somehow led to one conclusion: this kid is special. He's smart. He has leading guy potential.

Before he could even articulate the conclusion that there would be no mundane in this part of his life, Micah was applying it. When Micah's third-grade class was throwing an end-of-the-year party, he was not interested in attending. So, Micah got to stay home.

Micah had taken it to the next level with that particular scheme; apparently, his parents would believe anything he said. He had slowly been testing that, and it worked! This was how he lived his whole childhood – understanding his world and manipulating everyone to his advantage.

But he didn't tell anyone he knew these things. They would call him crazy. They would lock him up. Maybe that was supposed to happen too, but if that was the case, he wanted to prolong it if possible.

The first thing his parents would notice were his grades. Micah tried really hard not to pay attention to AP Calculus BC. Unfortunately, the material was intriguing as always, and that made it difficult not to absorb all of it. He had to resort to extremes; he pulled on an enormous headset and blasted the volume to immeasurable levels.

Nobody said anything. Because nothing important was allowed to happen in his life yet. That prematurely proved him right, but he wanted to finish what he started. When the math test came that Friday first period, he knew he was going to fail it. Micah was intentionally ill-prepared.

But when Micah saw the test, the first question was Describe the pattern: 1, 2, 1, 2. . .. They didn't get any harder after that. He turned in a blank paper with his name on it, but a week later, he got the test back with a note: Thanks for following instructions! You were the only person in class to notice, "Leave entire test BLANK for full credit." 100% This universe wasn't going to let him fail.

Micah moved on to the next phase of his experiment. He would break any rule he could think of. He uncaged nine penguins that were uncomfortably aware of their new climate and fled to Mr. Hoffman's classroom because he kept the thermostat at 53 degrees Fahrenheit. Nevertheless, there was silence in Micah's life for days after his actions. At last, on Wednesday, Mr. Hoffman approached him.

"Micah, it's time that we talked."

All at once, suspicions of his life being someone's story seemed ridiculous. He had been crazy for considering it. Then Mr. Hoffman finished what he was going to say.

"You can't chew gum in the hallways."

His experiment had reached a conclusion. He was not above the rules. And his life was real, not fiction.

"Not without giving me some!" Micah blinked and slid a piece of chewing gum into Mr. Hoffman's palm.

No, Micah thought. There was definitely something paranormal going on in his life.

He had pretty much already known it, but now it was confirmed by his scientific exploration.

Somewhere, not in this made-up universe, but in a real universe - there was an author, typing away onto his laptop computer. And that writer was typing the background story for him before he began his real adventure. It was why nothing happened unless it was essential to his characterization or to a distant storyline.

But Micah went home and lived life in routine. What was to be done? He was done with these experiments. Maybe there was more to discover, but it didn't matter, because there was nothing he could do about it.

Besides, he wasn't content with what he ended up discovering in the first place. He was an imagined image based off a series of sentences. His life was an illusion; it was worth nothing because he wasn't real. He wanted to be a real person more than anything else.

Micah was surfing the internet, pondering his consciousness. He wished there was something he could do to make himself feel better. It seemed absurd to him that there wasn't a place for someone like him to go, people who realized they were short story characters. If the author was going to cast him in this role, why was there no adventure? He couldn't even conjure a single thing that stuck out in this background story. Someone like him didn't deserve to be the main character of a story; even things were building up to something. And it truly didn't seem like they were.

His mother burst through his bedroom door. "Micah, Charles is at the door!"

He opened the front door. Charles was there with a skateboard, ready to "shred it." Micah was Charles' best friend, but Charles was not Micah's best friend. Now that he understood his existence a little better, Micah understood the situation. Since they were kids, Charles was pushed on him to be his best friend, and Micah never cared for him or his personality, but fate refused to hold back, and everything ended up this way.

It was the same with skateboarding. Micah used to be nonchalant about hating skateboarding, but since the revelation, he was ruthless. It didn't matter what he said about it, though. He wasn't supposed to know

31

anything about the frame his life hid in between, so nothing he said had any effect.

"Let's go to the park!" Charles exclaimed.

"No, thank you, Charles. I am too busy as well as not interested enough to go with you."

"I know, it's not as good as the one downtown, but our suburban skate park isn't too bad either!"

"I will shut the door now."

"Awesome! So, you got your safety gear ready?"

"I said no, Charles. . .."

"SPECTACULAR! We got to get a move on before the seniors take over, though!"

Micah sighed. He looked at the sky for guidance.

In a phenomenal instant, Micah thought of something incredible. Something that clicked.

He could be sure that he was just a story character. But it didn't matter he had friends, a good family, and he got lots of attention. He could do whatever he wanted and get away with it. Micah could do no wrong.

People in real life didn't get these privileges. Sure, times would always come that he wished to be something more, but most of the time, he was happy right where he was.

Micah went skateboarding with Charles that afternoon. It wasn't as bad as he thought it would be. He thought he might even end up liking it one day.

CHAPTER 6

Saleh

S aleh woke up to the warmth around him. He tried stretching, but he winced in pain. The last thing he could remember was being knocked off by an ice golem. Dariel twirled her fingers around his black hair as she nursed him back to health.

"You're up!" She said with excitement in her voice. Dariel had never seen a human and the idea of having one around totally fascinated her. She gave him soup and helped him sit up as he ate. Just then, Vulen stepped in with his catch for the day. His archery skills were second to none. He had a pout on his lips as he stared at Saleh who said hello to him almost immediately. He nodded his head as if observing his environment. Vulen was weary of humans. "Only Santa Claus is nice", he always argued. "He'll leave as soon as he is fine", Dariel said defensively without being asked.

Saleh got better as the days went by. One day, Dariel asked him, "Why were you in the mountains?" Dariel possessed so much calmness. Her beautiful hair glistened under the sun as he told her about his mission to save Faland. "Why do you stay here? I thought elves don't stay on mountains" Saleh asked innocently. "We're mountain elves" she replied sweetly. He told her a lot of things. His problems, the challenges he faced, and even told her about the plan with Gargoth, a huge man with a few strands of hair at the center of his head. Saleh excitedly talked about how great Gargoth was. Dariel looked at him with sadness on her face. "How did you kill the golem?" he asked as he was filled with curiosity. Dariel waved the question off by excusing herself. Saleh got well and wanted to leave the mountain top. He gave the elves a bag of gold coins, which they refused to take. "How do I reward you?" he asked. "Just keep yourself safe," Vulen said as he shot a bird with his arrow.

"You just can't leave yet!" Dariel said to him with concern written all over her. Her porcelain skin was so beautiful! It complemented her long, beautiful hair. "But why?" Saleh asked confusedly. "You have to learn to fight, to be safe and to protect yourself". "Dariel's Right!" Vulen added and paused "We wouldn't always be there to protect you," he said as he shrugged his shoulders and walked away. "To be a hero, there are lots of obstacles lots of monsters, but with knowledge on the right things, you'll prevail", Dariel said as she sewed.

Saleh made up his mind to stay and learn. Riches weren't enough for him, he just wanted to save Faland from all her oppressors. The goblins that ate the kids up, the one-eyed crows that invaded their farms, the heartless humans who took from the poor to enrich themselves all of them. The sun went down and Vulen asked Saleh to come with him to the woods, he taught him how to aim and shoot. Saleh was devoted and, soon, with so much practice, he was almost as good as Vulen.

Gorgoth was so excited because Saleh didn't return. e wore a gladiator sandal and went around bullying everyone. He was only nice because he wanted to deceive the town's savior Saleh into going away to the mountains so he can be killed by the dangerous creatures there.

Vulen and Saleh went to the woods to shoot. At noon, Dariel came with some snacks she made for them. For every aim that was hit on target, she divulged an important survival nugget to Saleh. "Trust no one", "Completely distinguish your enemies from your friends" "Never disclose your plans to anyone", she said to him firmly. Evening came and they retired home.

"I'll teach you magic and how to cast spells," Dariel said to him with a straight face. "But I can cast spells," Saleh said in defense. "That isn't

34

enough", Vulen said as he left the shelter. Dariel taught Saleh many magical tricks, improved his ability to cast spells. When you want to kill an enemy, look into his eyes and strike him in the heart. It rang like a bell in his ears.

Time passed and Saleh had to go. It was a sad goodbye. He had become part of them. They walked him to the end of the mountains and bade him farewell. "You can always come home," they said to him in unison. He nodded and a teardrop on his brown cheek. "Goodbye," he said and walked away occasionally looking back to see them again.

The whole town was in disarray. People ran helter-skelter. "Ghost!" some of them screamed locking their doors tightly as they saw Saleh. Gorgoth told them he was dead, and his corpse was eaten by vultures. Saleh felt so sad and went to see Gorgoth who was dining with the oppressors, he claimed to also dread. His face turned green and his mouth was agape. He didn't expect Saleh to return. "Come take this man to jail," Gandhi, one of the oppressors said to the soldiers and everyone burst into laughter.

At that spot, Saleh killed half of them with his bow and arrow staring deeply into their eyes. It took half of the soldiers to capture Saleh and put him behind bars. The night passed and morning came. Saleh wasn't in the cell. He was searched for but wasn't found. He had cast a spell on everyone there to sleep off as he magically took the keys out of the jailer's pocket. "I'll kill Gorgoth and hang his head on the city gates" he swore. He marched to Gorgoth's home. A defenseless Gorgoth appeared before him asking why he wasn't in jail. "Because I'm here to kill you", he replied. Gorgoth laughed hard and Saleh looked at Gorgoth in his eyes and struck an arrow to his chest.

Everyone around ran in fear. He took a sword from the guards and cut Gorgoth's head off. The news spread and all the bad people fled in fear. Gorgoth's head was embalmed and placed on the city gate. The people cheered in excitement and crowned Saleh king. Occasionally, he visited

the elves and took to them a lot of food. Saleh felt fulfilled. Faland was
happy and peaceful ever after.

CHAPTER 7

A Bargain

Magda hadn't considered the weather reports when she made her way into the woods that day. The weather had been sunny, and the temperatures had been rather mild all week long. Why should that suddenly change just because I've got errands to do outside? She wondered to herself as she grumbled about the rain clouds that were rolling in overhead.

As the clouds muddied the blue sky above, Magda remained determined to complete the tasks that had sent her out to the woods. She would get the photo she needed for her photography class. Marlon had told her not to bother taking the photography class, as he deemed it a waste of money. He said that Magda never finished anything she ever set herself to and that there wasn't any reason to expect that this endeavor of becoming a photographer to be any different than her failed ventures into pottery, woodworking, painting, and macramé.

Out of spite, Magda signed up for the classes, which had begun in August of that year. She had attended every single class, completed every single assignment, gone above and beyond to learn more about it in her spare time, and had shown Marlon that she meant to prove him wrong on this one. Marlon, of course, didn't care about it one way or the other. He just wanted Magda to find something that would fill her time and make her happy. If that thing happened to be taking photos just to spite him, he figured that worked just well enough.

As Magda got deeper into the woods, the trees seemed to drink in every bit of light that streamed in from the sky, leaving very little for the forest floor below. In spite of the terrible conditions this created for photography, and in spite of Magda's comprehensive understanding of how lighting worked, she pressed on, looking for the perfect scene to shoot. She had seen it days before but hadn't had her camera with her. She told herself that she had only been scouting and that there was no need to bring her camera with her. In retrospect, she realized that she should have brought the camera so she could capture that moment.

She had found a small, unique grouping of mushrooms in the forest that had a unique, seemingly purposeful formation among them. They were arranged in a perfect circle and the odds of this, Magda thought, were slim to none! She had to get her camera and come back for a photo. For all she knew now, however, deer or other woodland creatures had come by and eaten the mushrooms. For all she knew, they could have been trampled by an unknowing moose traveling through the wood. Still, she pressed onward to the area where she had remembered seeing them.

As she approached the area where she had remembered seeing them just a couple of days previously, she held her breath. She wasn't sure how she would react if they were no longer in the place where she had last seen them, but she knew that Marlon would see the brunt of her anger about the situation. He wouldn't have really been to blame for whatever had eaten or trampled them, nor would he be to blame for her neglecting to bring her camera when she had come scouting earlier in the week. He would, however, be responsible for getting under her skin, but that was a badge of honor she knew he would proudly wear. For that, she would hold this whole ordeal against him until he soothed her with forehead kisses and hot chocolate.

She crested a small mound in the woods and breathed a sigh of relief. The mushrooms were still there, and they looked as fresh and bright as they had when she came to scout. There was something alluring about those mushrooms and the formation in which they grew. She snapped her shot and marveled at how perfectly her camera captured their likeness. She failed to remember the looming clouds overhead and that there should not have been ample light in these woods to so beautifully capture the mushrooms in that way. She saw nothing odd about the light that flowed seemingly from nowhere to illuminate her shot.

"Beautiful shot," a delicate voice came from the branch above her head. Magda's head shot up to find a rather diminutive woman sitting on the branch.

"Oh, thank you. I'm sorry, I didn't see you there before."

"I didn't mean to startle you. May I see your shot?" Magda slowly held the camera out to the woman in the tree. It wasn't until Magda's camera was in the woman's hands that Magda realized how impossibly tiny this woman really was. The camera sat in her lap in much the same way that a child might hold a gentleman's briefcase. The woman commented on the composition of her shot, the lighting, and the angle.

"You really know your stuff, Magda. Great work. I'm sure Mr. Yamashida will be impressed with it." Magda's blood ran cold. How could this impossibly tiny woman know her name, the name of her photography instructor, or that this shot was for an assignment? The trepidation and alarm must have been plain on Magda's face.

"You're not as quiet as you think, wandering through these woods. All I had to do was listen for about five minutes before I felt like I was a part of your world." Magda heaved a sigh.

"Oh, man. I didn't even realize I was talking. I'm so sorry." She chuckled at herself, taking the camera back from the woman and setting about returning the device to it carrying case.

"I'm Saoirse, by the way."

"It's nice to meet you, S... Saoi—"

"Saoirse. It's okay, it's an Irish Gaelic name that's hard to pronounce." Magda nodded, a little embarrassed.

"So, do you spend a lot of time in trees?" Saoirse giggled to herself.

"You could say that I do, yeah. Do you spend a lot of time cursing in the woods?"

"You could say that I do, yeah." Magda and Saoirse laughed. "I like to scout for photo locations in places where nature is more present than man. I find that I capture the best photos in locations like that."

"Ah, yes. Nature has a lot of beauty to offer, indeed."

"I'm so grateful I got here when I did," Magda said, looking down at the mushrooms. "The light is so dim here now. I wouldn't have been able to get nearly as good a shot in this light."

"I thought that might be the case. I added a little more lighting from up here when you were lining up your shot. I didn't want you to have to hold today against... Marlon, was it?" Magda laughed again at her unwitting oversharing.

"Yes, Marlon it was. Thank you for that. What did you use?" Magda looked around but saw no equipment.

"Oh, a little of this, a little of that. My question is, what would you give me in return for that perfect shot?" Saoirse kept a cool smirk on her face as she maintained eye contact with Magda, who froze. She hadn't expected to end up in debt to someone she didn't know, for a favor she didn't ask them to do for her.

"I'm not sure... What did you have in mind?"

"Well, I was wondering if you might help me find my way back out of the woods? I'm quite small, as you can see, and I'm a little bit worried something might nip me by the scruff and carry me off." Magda raised her eyebrows.

"Oh, certainly. I can show you out. Do you need a ride to the main road?"

"You know, that would be lovely. Help me out of this tree, would you love?" Saoirse lifted her arms so Magda could take hold of her like a

40

small child. As Magda guided her safely to the ground, she marveled at the size of this woman. She really was the size of an infant, with the proportions of a woman. It was baffling. Perhaps some form of dwarfism with very little proportion disparity, she thought.

Just as Saoirse's feet hit the ground, she took hold of Magda's wrists and began speaking a language Magda didn't understand. Immediately. Magda's knees buckled and she was crouched in the center of the circle, arms outstretched and held in place by the tiny creature. Saoirse's eyes glowed as she spoke English once again.

"It's nothing personal, Magda. I just needed a way out and you were in the right place at the right time." Magda felt her very essence sliding out of her body. It seemed nearly like a phantom limb phenomenon when she swore that she could feel Saoirse's essence seeping into her body where hers had just been. Suddenly, the world seemed massive.

Magda's body stood up before her, looking at her hands, breathing in deeply and making strange motions with her hands.

"No magic. I'm free." Saoirse, now in Magda's body, looked down at Magda. "Thank you. I know you will hate me for this, but please know that you have my sincerest, undying gratitude." At this, she grabbed the camera bag and ran out of the woods toward Magda's car.

Magda, now in Saoirse's tiny body, ran as quickly as she could to keep up with the body that had just been stolen from her.

"Wait! Come back!" She was still yards away when the car rumbled to life and lurched as the driver tried to figure out how to make it work. She kept running, feeling the burning in her lungs as she did so.

Just as she reached the road where her car was parked, it was as though she slammed into a thick pane of unyielding glass with full force. She bounced off the barrier and fall onto her bottom. Her car sped off, leaving her in these woods forever.

Magda had never meant to trade her whole life for the perfect shot.

41

CHAPTER 8

The Genius

Tonight, we are going to witness the power of the human mind. An extraordinary existence that lies within you and the power within it has so much untapped potential. We are going to tap into that genius potential to give you the most relaxing and serene peace that your body and mind have ever experienced. First, you must clear your mind. Let's do this with an organizational approach. Imagine a room; it can be stark white, it can be an ordinary office; maybe it's a storage room, or an extraterrestrial room that is dark with sleek modern touches. This room will be your way to file and organize your thoughts, putting them away for the night.

Let us start collecting those thoughts, by exploring your thought superhighway and gathering everything we can find. Collect the thoughts however you need; if they are organized maybe you can set up a roadblock. Position yourself to slow, then halt the thoughts, processing which way they need to go. Compressing the thoughts into tiny manageable pieces. Maybe your thoughts are scattered, you can lay a net or a trap, and gather them all up at once? Then take each thought, figure out what it is, assign it to a file. As all the thoughts ramble and bounce around in your mind, stop them and gather them into a pile. Maybe some thoughts are linked together, place them within the same file or box; however big you need that storage bin or containment system to be. Your stack is growing higher and higher as all the thoughts from the day leave your thought highway and go into your manageable file system.

Once you have a hefty pile, you lift it up. The weight feeling like a burden and weighing you down, you take the thoughts to your organizational room. Let's begin filing away these thoughts. Stacking them, filing them, whatever you need to do to clean up your mind space. Making things nice, tidy, and neat. Take your time, go through every thought, making sure it is tucked away, not going to fall off and ramble its way back onto the thought highway. If you feel any loose thoughts escaping, making their way back onto the thought highway, let it go, don't fight it. Finish putting away what you have now, these thoughts are ready to be put to rest. Once everything is put in its place, go back to the highway for a last sweep. Any errant thoughts can be grabbed up now. Catch those thoughts and take them back to the organization room. Are all your thoughts tucked away? If yes, your mind is blank and ready to explore? If no, take a moment and keep collecting and storing until you're ready to move on.

You leave the organization room behind you now. You travel through your mind; we're going to tap into the parts you do not use often enough. You can visualize your brain, the parts you use often are alive and electric. As you pass these parts by, allow them to calm down. Let them rest, they have done enough for today, we don't need them for what we are going to do. You pass by the central part, the one that controls your breathing, you heart rate, gently caress it. Let it know it can relax too, it can slow down. Feel your breathing calm, your heart rate a soft cadence; the reassurance that life is within you and will continue to be so in the morning. As you feel your mind relaxing you continue to travel through. Passing the parts, you do not use enough, seeing them with their soft warm glow, welcoming you to tap into them. Once you have located the untapped potential, touch it. Reach up your arms and stretch them long. Stretch your torso and back, twist to reach it. Make your legs long all the way to your toes. Now you feel it, you're touching this dull area and a warm sensation is starting to come alive and you can feel it washing over you. It starts to warm up and emit a little happy glow that travels all through your body. Your muscles start to relax as the warmness caress it, your mind feels pleasant, bubbling and cloudy, until it sinks into the warm, soft light, then you can see a vivid green field all around you.

The sky is blue, the tall grass, soft and green. Your entire body feels warm and relaxed. Let's see if this is the true potential of your mind with a little test. Imagine yellow dandelions growing all over the field. Big ones, small ones. Count them as you add the yellow dandelions, until you can't count. There's too many, millions and millions of yellow flowers surrounding you with happiness and joy. This is the power of your mind, if your mind isn't cooperating then you're not ready for this area. Don't give up, go back, explore your brain, find another untapped area and keep trying. You will find one that will let you explore. Once you're in a warm area and you see the field that you can control, you are there. Now that we are all there let's practice this new and pleasing sensation of control, turn the dandelions into to their fluffy white flowers, ready to release their seeds into the world. All around you, in a field full of white fluffy dandelions. Pick one up. Take a deep breath in, then blow it out slowly. Watching the seeds spiral from the flower into the air. As the seeds float back to the earth, steady yourself. This is just a very small power that rests inside you, it can do so much more. Take another deep breath in as you pick another dandelion. Exhale as you blow those seeds and come to terms with the fact you are a genius. You are capable of anything you set your mind to. Rest and relaxation can help you tap into that genius.

You command your mind and body. Right now, you command them to relax. Your entire body is soft, relaxed, and pliable. Your mind is warm, enriched, and welcoming to the thoughts of your tapped genius potential. You can go anywhere in the world right now, without leaving this state of relaxation. Where do you want to go? Picture that place; is it an ocean shore, a busy city, a small village, or a place you know well? What does it smell like? What can you hear? What can you see? How does it make you feel? Take a moment and enjoy this place, explore the sensations. Is it everything you hoped it would be?

44

This is your mind allowing you to experience the most wonderful sensations whenever you want it to. This power is incredible. You want to be on a beach in Greece, done. You want to be in the mountains in Asia, done. You want to be anywhere in space or time, you can do that. You are a wonderful, amazing creature, with limitless abilities as you bring yourself into ultimate relaxation at the same time. Would you like to see what else your mind is capable of?

Picture the tallest building in the world. Now get to the top of it. How does your mind get you there? Do you instantly appear on the top of the building? Do you walk up to the building, enter, and take an elevator? Do you start the arduous task of climbing the stairs? Do you gear up and climb the side of the building? Or maybe you come from above, using a parachute as you fall from a plane to land on top of the tallest building in the world. So many possibilities can spring from one simple suggestion. If you can get to the top of this building, then you can do anything. Take your time, or get it done quickly. It doesn't matter, because all the potential to do it, is inside your mind.

Can you understand now how beautiful and creative your mind is? Your mind can grow and continue to astound you every day, if you let it. Listen to your mind, let it guide you... Let your mind connect with your heart, picture the direct link between the two. This connection will know what you want the most in this life. Do not stop it, do not slow it down. Let it carry you away, showing you your hopes and dreams and how you can achieve them. Stay in this state of relaxation, do not let the errant thoughts break out of their storage room. They are locked away, stored nice and neatly for tomorrow. Tonight, is not about any of those thoughts, quickly lock that door, then forget it. It is about you, who you are, what you want, and how you are going to get it.

Everything becomes clear and easy to manage. Just like organizing your thoughts, your mind can control and process anything you bring its way. Let it take over, just as it took you into this deep relaxation. Once you are in total control of your mind, then you can shut it down and go to sleep. Enjoy your peaceful rest, and I look forward to seeing your genius potential in the world.

CHAPTER 9

Connecting with Nature

And there was a lady who enjoyed going out camping, she enjoyed her own company, she enjoyed peace and solitude, she enjoyed being one with nature and felt that being one with nature and being out camping on your own helped to connect with the world around you. Helped to keep you grounded. And so, she decided to go out camping and with her backpack on her back she trekked out into the countryside, trekked through woodland, enjoying the sounds of the birds, hearing a woodpecker at a tree, the sound of a distant stream, the sounds of rustling leaves as the wind blows a breeze. The sound of each footstep, the smells in the woods and occasionally she would touch a branch of a tree to feel that connection, to feel the sensations of the bark on her fingertips. She would stop and watch butterflies dancing around flowers and the way beams of light would dance through the canopies above. And she appreciated the reduced sound that you get in the woods, the way everything just seems so much more peaceful and calmer.

And after some time, walking through the woods, she found herself reaching a gate, passing through that gate and entering into a vast meadow with hills either side, deer off in the distance, just grazing and watching out. She could see birds flying overhead and other animals in the meadow and all the different wildflowers. And she set up a camp, up on the hillside, overlooking the meadow. Able to look one way to the woodland, able to look the other way further down into the meadow, all the way down to the lake way off in the distance. And she prepared her area and created a campfire and set up a tent and then sat down just inside that tent in front of the campfire, listening to the crackling fire as the fire began to burn down until it was just giving off heat, no flames, just glowing embers by nightfall. And as the sun set, so she began to hear and notice bats flying overhead catching insects and just the calming sounds of the outdoors. And she could feel the warmth of the fire as she sat just inside her tent having something to eat. And she enjoyed this experience, she valued this experience, of being able to look up and see the stars across the sky, of noticing the way the firelight makes shadows dance and seems almost hypnotic as you gaze at it.

And as she sat there gazing at the fire she started eating an apple, enjoying the sweetness of the apple. Valuing the way that the apple was created with its skin to hold the goodness in. And then she noticed that it was starting to rain a bit. And she had camped in all conditions and she liked it when it rained. She felt it calming and comforting. So, she backed into her tent, climbed into her sleeping bag, zipped up the entrance to the tent, she knew her tent was well and truly grounded, safe and secure. And at first, she could hear large drops of water hitting the fabric of the tent and she had a light on inside the tent, just hanging above her and she could notice the drops of rain hitting the tent and those drops started large and infrequent and gradually started to get more frequent as the rain got heavier outside. And she knew that the rain would put the fire out and as she was approaching bedtime anyway she wasn't going to need the fire. She was plenty warm enough in her sleeping bag in her tent. And she just rested back in that sleeping back, felt all snuggly, warm and cozy. Just listening to the way, the rain bounced on the tent. The way the wind made the sides of the tent move and she found it so calming, so relaxing. A bit like sitting in a conservatory on a rainy day or sitting in a car on a rainy day. Just being able to listen to that rain while keeping dry and warm and comfortable.

And she relaxed back listening to the rain and found that the rain was rhythmically guiding her asleep. And although she was attempting to keep her attention focused on the rain, on enjoying the sound of the rain, her eyes would flicker and she would find that she kept dropping off asleep for a moment at a time, until she totally fell asleep deeply and comfortably. And the next thing she knew, she woke up in the morning feeling so refreshed and revitalized, to the sounds of birds and morning animals announcing the morning. She opened the tent and saw the sunlight and breathed in the fresh air that seemed even more fresh, as if the rain had washed any pollutants out of the air. She could see the morning dew across the meadow, across the plants, see some of it turning to mist as the sun continued to rise. And she climbed out of the tent, stretched herself and then went and prepared herself for the morning, restarted the fire, to make herself some breakfast and a cup of tea, boiled a pot of water and just loved that moment when the pot would start whistling to let her know that she is ready to poor the tea and that feeling of drinking a tea in the countryside out of a flask cup or a camping cup, rather than a typical mug at home. Something about holding that cup in her hands, feeling the warmth of that tea.

And she just sat back and enjoyed the view, enjoyed looking down towards the lake, enjoyed looking over to the woodland, enjoyed watching the birds in the sky. And she knew the grass was still slightly damp from the night before, but if it wasn't for that, you would almost not have realised that it had rained. Because of the fact that there were no clouds in the sky, everything was just blue in every direction. And the air was fresh and cool and she could feel it in her nostrils, feel it on her skin and she rested there, drinking a tea, enjoying a moments peace and solitude, enjoying this time inside her mind, with her own thoughts and ideas about nature, about what there is to enjoy in life, to look forward to in life, to appreciate in life. As she gazed down at the meadow and she thought it was curious how every single blade of grass is actually unique and different to every other single blade of grass, yet at a glance, you could just assume that all those blades of grass are just a blade of grass looking like any other blade of grass and it is only when you get down to each blade and truly and honestly take a close look at each blade of grass that you notice that each one is slightly different to each other one and yet all of that difference doesn't take away from the beauty of the meadow, the harmony of the meadow, the way everything seems

49

connected, the way everything seems to have a purpose out here in the country and she enjoyed her little insights like this.

Like the sadness of a predator catching its prey and yet had the predator not caught the prey, it wouldn't have turned out so well for the predator or the predator's offspring. Or the joy when the prey gets away and how that turns out well for the prey's offspring. And how everything, from the blades of grass to the deer, to the birds of prey, how everything is connected in a balance. And she is just an observer on this. And she enjoyed having thoughts like this, thoughts that allowed her to connect, to understand deeper meaning and to have an appreciation for the world around her. She could almost feel the countryside in her heart, as if she was one, in-step, in rhythm, in harmony with the countryside, with the world around her. Able to just enjoy being in the moment. Not trapped in the past in her mind, worrying about other things, not trapped in the future in her mind, worrying about what might be, but enjoying being in the here and now, accepting that what is, is. And just enjoying what she can do here and now.

And during the day, as the sun grows higher, she kept her camp set up, she wandered away from her camp, she wandered down the hill, she wandered through the meadow down towards the lake, she walked all the way to the lake and barefooted she walked in to the lake, just a little way in, to feel the water, to feel the coolness of the water on her feet as it flowed and lapped gently on the shore. And gazed down through that water at small fish swimming around her feet, tickling her toes, darting out of the way whenever she moved her feet and then coming back again when her feet were stationary. And she just stood there with her eyes closed, breathing in and out, the fresh air, the way the air smelled even fresher over the water, enjoying the way the sun glistened on the lake, the way the breeze blew across the lake. Enjoyed the peace and silence here. With no-one else around, just her in nature. Able to connect, no worries, no phones, no distractions, just a connection with the environment.

And through the day she wandered around the lake, sat by the lake, meditated, took in the environment and felt a connection with the environment. She had something to eat at lunch time and then as it approached the end of the day she went back to her tent to settle down for another night. And again, she lit a fire, just for some light and a bit of warmth in the evening and to cook some food with. And she had something to eat in the evening, listened to the cracking fire, felt its warmth, enjoyed the way that shadows danced, the flames flickered, as that fire gradually burned down to just embers. And then when she was ready and felt it was time to sleep, she moved back into the tent, zipped up the entrance, laid down in her sleeping bag and just listened to the evening sounds outside. And as she listened to those evening sounds outside, so she began to breathe deep comfortable breaths, with each exhalation being longer than each inhalation, having a sense of a connection with the world around her, focusing on her breathing and other sounds around her, as she began to drift comfortably asleep and as she drifted comfortably asleep so she drifted into some comfortable dreams for the night and she knew she was going to enjoy those dreams, before waking in the morning feeling so calm and refreshed, to enjoy another day on this hillside and in this valley and she knew she was going to spend a few more days out here, exploring and enjoying being one with nature before deciding to take down her tents and head back to normality. But she was going to make the most of her time here first and she thought all that as she drifted comfortably, relaxed, asleep.

CHAPTER 10

The Mountain

You are sitting atop a mountain, and you are as big as the mountain. You don't know who you are, or what you are, or how you got there, but you are gigantic, and you are, here, on earth, larger than life.

You place your hand down and cup the peak of the mountain next to you. It feels so strange to hold an entire mountain in your hand.

The trees on the mountain comprise merely fuzz, which pleasantly tickles your skin. Out of curiosity, you bend your head down and lick the mountain, just to see what these tiny, miniscule trees feel like on your tongue.

It is like licking algae, and, with it, the earth sends this loving kiss back up to you, electricity from the core sparking through the conduit of your saliva into your brain.

By being so large, over all the familiar foliage of the earth, its power affects you in a way that it never has before, for you are able to experience so much of it at once, and, as it is put into perspective by your new size and stature, you are humbled by its infinite nature, the way it spreads, over the mountains, as the mountains spread over the land, with no end in sight.

The mountains get bigger and bigger the farther they spread, and some of them are so big you cannot see over them. Still, you know, you could climb past them with ease. And so, you will. You stand up and are immediately thrown out of whack by the height your head reaches once your body is fully extended into the sky.

To your utmost surprise, you nearly can see over the highest peaks, and, as you do, you see the glow of the moon behind them, a great bright light, and your curiosity to come over them grows. You look down and see a few rivers, besides you, flowing down past you, and behind you. You reach your finger down and, gently, with your tip, feel the flow of the water.

Your finger is so large that it cannot fit in the river, and you do not want to disrupt the size and path of the river, so you just get a very brief feel with the utmost tip of your skin. It is beautiful. You take a deep breath and allow yourself to get acclimated with your size.

The winds are rushing at your head and stiller towards the ground, the atmosphere changes multiple times over the length of your body you are so large.

You feel as if you are nearly in space, but only really just barely touching the clouds.

Once you feel comfortable, you take steps, very gently, so as to intrude as little as possible on the small-scale intricate natural landscapes happening all around you, beneath you.

In a few steps, you are there, at the highest peaks.

You place your hands on them and peak through, and there you see it, the human landscape. Cities, as far as the eye can see, lights, in the darkness of the night, calm and serene, asleep, and so very small.

You are amazed.

How will this experience be, now, as you are? You will go down into the towns, you must, and you must feel them in this new light.

So you travel through the peaks, climbing over them like climbing over a small fence, and make your way down, through the range, the mountains becoming smaller and smaller, until a couple of careful steps later, being very, very quiet so as not to disturb the encroaching city, you are at the foothills.

It is breathtaking.

A small lake nearby is sitting tranquil in the night, the moonlight glowing off of it.

It is incredible to see the entire thing in one eyeful, all the trees around it, so small, so serene. You keep going, off into the city.

The city is asleep, totally. As if by chance, there is no one outside to see you, no one to witness this great, grand giant who has come to see, to put life into a new perspective, a giant who, at some time, might've lived in such a city, in another life, so long ago, before he grew, and incarnated, here, to exist as this giant being, watching over.

For what it's worth, the city is serene from up here.

In a way that may not be perceptible when you are lost in its maze, there is an intricacy and a quaintness to the seeming complexities of human living that take a certain simple pattern from the right vantage, from far away, from the sky, almost as if taking a cue from the eye of the heavens.

There is an order amongst the chaos, and there is a shape to the concrete jungle that is recognizable from a great distance. Journeying over the city, it ends very soon, and, here you are again, before a great empty abyss, this time a long patch of plains.

You look back, and see the mountains, like looking across a small room, across the city, barely any distance has been travelled, it feels, in this form, yet you know, millions of lives have been passed over, still sleeping, peacefully, behind you.

You progress over the plains, and, it occurs to you, soon you will be upon a beach, and an ocean. Sporadic spurts of life come and go beneath you, all very, very, quiet, and all asleep.

Farms, and windmills, and little silos, tiny dirt roads with fuzz vibrating off them, flowing little hairs of stalks forming together into one mass like individuals' threads sewn into tiles on an intricate quilt. You keep going, and, even in your gigantic form, the expanse hypnotizes you in its seemingly infinite being.

Land, going on, such long stretches at a time, the world so large, even here, yet so much smaller than it has ever seemed. What will occur at the ocean? What will it feel like to stand on the shore? Soon, you will find out. The foliage begins to break up, and you can see the shore in the great distance.

You are approaching. A great wind blows the air of the sea into your face, and you are transported back to another place and time, a small child, at the beach, gazing out at the horizon, wondering what infinite wonders await.

And, here you are, now, however you came to be here, this large, prepared to take that voyage, and wander into the ocean for yourself, to see what's there. The beach itself is about the length of your foot.

If you didn't purposefully rub your foot against the sand, you might have missed it and gone straight into the waters.

You are taken aback at the thought of how absolutely tiny the grains of the sand on the beach must be to you now, like molecules, or atoms, you cannot even perceive them.

You place both feet on the beach, and stand for a second, just taking in the grandeur of the sight before you.

Oddly, at this size, gazing out at the horizon from the beach, even though the beach is just a small sliver to you, is no different than gazing out at it from any other size, for it itself is so infinite, so huge, that it is still endless, in this size or another. You still cannot see anything but deep, dark blue, stretching out to the very edges of the planet. You take an incredibly deep breath, and you step out, into the water.

With your first step, the water barely submerges the bottom of your foot, and then, with the second step, your foot is submerged, then you are at your knees, then your waist, then for a while you are just half away in, walking along the bottom of the ocean, swaying slowly in the water.

Whales and sharks swim all around you, you know, but you cannot feel them, or, at least, have not yet. They are like tadpoles to you, keeping their distance.

You keep going and get a little tiny bit deeper with each step. After a while, you look back at where you came from, and realize you cannot see land. Then you look all around you and realize there is no land visible anywhere.

However far away any land may be, it is not visible. You keep going forward, the way you were going. Eventually, your chest is in the water, and the water is almost up to your neck. You must've been walking for several hours now.

You take a minute to pause and just exist in this water. It is the most relaxing and awe-inspiring situation you have ever experienced.

You lay on your back and float around in the water, infinity before you at all sides, infinity below, infinity above, infinity everywhere, surrounding you.

You continue on through the ocean, and into your view come a glowing spot of land, in the distance.

You begin walking towards it and notice that you are coming out of the water, slowly at first, then faster, until the water is back at your ankles, and then, with one more step, you are on land. This land is unrecognizable to you, not that it would be.

This is some island, somewhere, far, far off the coast of wherever you came from. There is obviously no human life on the island.

It is untouched.

There is only you, and whatever wilderness happens to be occurring naturally.

You are a little cold from coming out of the water, the raging winds of the atmosphere coming against your wet skin, so you decide to get down closer to the ground.

You kneel down, and pat your hands around, feeling the land.

There are many, many trees, and much, much foliage, and so the land is very soft, velveteen, padded and comfortable, and it feels very warm to you now.

You decide to lay your whole body down on this land, and you curl up, and look out, with your hand lying on your head, folded up, as in a fetal position, into the ocean.

You watch the swaying of the ocean and become hypnotized by the dancing of the moonlight reflected off the water, and the movement of the water itself.

Your eyelids become heavy and start to fall.

As they close, the sound of the ocean around you intensifies, and, again, you are taken back to another place, much smaller, in your mind, dwarfed, even in your size, by the immense infinity of the ocean, and the land, and the earth.

The sounds are gigantic, much more so than you, and they go on forever, and ever, and they never end, perpetuating on past your sleeping body.

CHAPTER 11

A Snowman Saves Christmas

Once upon a time there was a snowman who lived in the Christmas wonderland high on a hill in a house sitting on a tree. It was not a tree house. It was a real house in a tree. It was normal in the Christmas Wonderland. There were also gingerbread houses, huge Christmas trees and much more fantastic.

But let's get back to our snowman, whose biggest wish was to be a Christmas elf. However, only elves were allowed to be Christmas Elves. It was written in the big Christmas book.

Nevertheless, the snowman tried it year after year. He disguised himself once as elf to get into the magnificent Christmas factory. But he already noticed the guard on the gate. Maybe his carrot had betrayed him on the face? Or maybe he was just more spherical than anyone else.

It would work this year. Because the snowman had a great idea. He wanted to pack presents himself and distribute them to the children. But could Santa not be angry with him? And he could finally conjure the longed-for smile into the faces of the children.

First, the gifts had to come from. But where to take and not steal? He had to make some money somehow. But what should he do? He sleds incredibly well on the sled. But you could not earn money with that.

He remembered something. He slid happily and started to make little snowballs. Then he took a sign and sat down in the snow. On the sign it was written: "Every Ball 3 Taller". That would have to work. Everyone likes snowball fights. But the snowman was sitting in vain hour after hour. Nobody even bought a snowball.

So, he asked the blacksmith if he could help. He only laughed loudly. "What do you want to help me with?" The blacksmith asked. "If you stand by the fire with me, you'll melt. Do you want to serve me as drinking water? "

"That's right." Thought the snowman. It had to be something cold. So he went to the ice factory. There large blocks of ice were made to build igloos. But even here, the snowman was laughed at. "How do you want to help me?" Asked the factory manager. "The blocks are so heavy, if you want to push them, break your thin stick sleeves."

"That's right." Thought the snowman again. It has to be something where it's cold and the work is not too hard. So, the snowman went to the ice cream seller. He was taken with the idea and said: "You are certainly a good ice cream seller! You're never too cold, and if ice is missing for cooling, we'll just take something from you. "When the snowman heard that, he was startled. "Ice cream from me?" He asked. "I think I was wrong in the door," he said and walked quickly away.

Now the snowman was sad. Nothing he tried worked. He sank to the ground in the middle of the city. His hat slipped over his sad button eyes. He picked up his violin and played a Christmas carol. That always helped him when he was sad.

As he played, he was so lost in thought that he did not notice the passing people throwing him some change. Only when a stranger passed in said: "A wonderful Christmas carol. That's one of my favorites. Keep playing snowman. "He listened.

He pushed his hat up and saw the change in front of him. "That's money!" He said softly. And played on. "That's money!" He shouted loudly and kept playing. He grinned all over his face and sang with his heart's content: "Tomorrow children will give something. Tomorrow we will be happy ... "

With the newly earned money, he bought gifts and wrapping paper. A doll there and a car here. Hardworking was packed and laced. And the cord passed through the hole. "One right, one left - yes the snowman comes and brings it!"

But wait. How should the presents reach the children from here? The snowman considered. "I can not wear it. But I do not have a Christmas sleigh either. And Santa will hardly lend me his. Besides, the reindeer would want to eat my carrot. "

The snowman could sled incredibly well on a sledge, but it was not always just mountain off. So what to do? Again, the snowman had a great idea. He tied the presents to a snail. Snails can carry a lot. That would work.

Just when he was done, a Christmas elf passed by. "What will that be when it's done?" The Christmas elf asked. The snowman stood proudly next to his snail. "This is my Christmas slug! And I'm giving presents to the children this year. "

The Christmas elf looked at the snowman and the snail in wonderment. "I would laugh now, if it were not so sad," he said then. "You know that a snail is way too slow to deliver gifts to all the children in the world? I mean, she herself would be too slow to supply just this village. "

The happy grin passed by the snowman and the elf continued: "In addition, unfortunately, these are not enough gifts. You would need a million billion more. But it does not matter anyway. Anyway, Christmas is out this year! "

When the snowman heard that, he no longer understood the world. "Christmas is out? That does not work! "The Christmas elf nodded:" And if that works. Santa Claus got sick and can not distribute presents. "

"Naaaein", the snowman breathed in astonishment and looked at the elf in disbelief. "Santa Claus can not get sick." The Christmas elf nodded again: "That's right. Usually not. But this year it's so cold that even our Christmas elves are too cold. "The snowman got nervous:" But

60

Christmas, so Christmas ... so, what about Christmas? "He ran around hectic and talked to himself:" No, no, no, no, that can not be. A Christmas without presents is not a Christmas. "

The Christmas elf interrupted the snowman. "Christmas is very Christmas without gifts. The presents were getting more and more and almost too much over the last few years anyway. "The snowman collapsed briefly and breathed out," Yeah, yaaaaaaaaaa, that's alright. "Then he stood straight up and said," But with presents it's a lot more beautiful."

The Christmas elf shook his head: "Christmas is the festival of charity. No need for presents. "The snowman whirled around and said quietly," Yes, that's right. "Then he took one of his presents and held it up to the Christmas elf's nose." But look how beautiful the presents are. With such a gift, I can show my charity much better than without. "

Then he let the gift disappear behind his back and looked at the Christmas elf sadly. "Look, now it's gone. Is not that sad? Imagine the many little sad googly eyes standing in front of a Christmas tree, under which there are no presents. And now tell the children that we do not need presents, because Christmas is the feast of charity! "

The Christmas elf said, "Okay, maybe you're right. But what should we do? It's too cold! "The snowman tossed the gift aside and slid to the Christmas elf:" Ha! Exactly! It's too cold! ... for Santa Claus. But I'm a snowman! "Then he turned in a circle and began to sing:" I'm never too cold, I'll be so old. I can hurry and hurry, distribute gifts to children. All you have to do is help me with stuff and team. Take me to Santa Claus quickly. "

The Christmas elf covered its ears: "Now stop singing. I'll take you there already. "The snowman jumped in the air with joy:" Juhu! Hey, that was almost rhyming. You could also sing a song. "And so, the snowman talked a long while on the way to Santa - to the chagrin of the Christmas Elf.

61

Arrived at Santa Claus, he was very surprised to see a snowman at home. Usually there were only Christmas elves. But Santa Claus loved the idea that Christmas should not be canceled. Because he was of the opinion that Christmas is simply nicer with gifts. But how should the snowman distribute so many presents?

The snowman chewed nervously on his lips. He was so close to living his biggest dream. "We do not have to distribute all presents," he said. "Everyone gets a little less this year. It's still better than nothing, is not it? "Santa looked at the snowman:" I do not think that's a bad idea. That should work! But how do you want to drive the presents? You can not have my sled! "

The snowman was on the verge of despair. "Only solve this one problem and my dream comes true." He thought. Then he said sheepishly, "Well, I'm a pretty good sledger!" And looked questioningly at Santa. The Christmas elf intervened: "Oh, that's all nonsense! Then you only supply the children who live at the bottom of a mountain? Or how should I imagine that? "

But Santa raised his hand and moved his fingers as if he were scratching the air. Out of nowhere a huge snow slide emerged under the snowman. Then Santa said, "You're such a good sledger. This snow mountain will accompany you. He is a never-ending snow slope. So, you can go sledding anywhere. "

The snowman looked at the huge snow mountain and said: "That .... Is ... "he suddenly jumped in the air and shouted loudly:" ... the hammer! Sledding! That's not what I imagined in my wildest dreams. "

The snowman was happy as never before. But Santa raised his index finger again and said admonishingly: "But watch out by the fireplaces! I've burnt my butt once before! "But the snowman let it go cold:" Oh, I have so much snow, if I burn my butt, I'll just make a new one - haha. "Then he grinned at Santa, jumped on his sled and was gone.

And so, the snowman saved Christmas, which was way too cold, but just right for the snowman!

CHAPTER 12

The Little Field Mouse Learns Magic

It was a lovely, balmy summer day. The little field mouse and her friends played the whole day in the field by the pond. They played catching, hiding and ran to the bet.

Suddenly the little field mouse said to her friends, "Do you know what, now I'll conjure something for you!" The friends looked at each other in astonishment. "You can do magic?" They sat on a recumbent tree trunk and watched the little field mouse in their preparations. This curled up a small stump and spread a cloth over it. On the other hand, she put a cylinder on the cloth and covered it with another cloth.

Then she raised her paws up: "Abera ca Dabera." And it happened ... nothing. The friends looked a little disappointed. The little field mouse pulled the cloth from the cylinder with a "Wusch" and reached in with his left hand. At the same time, she reached down with her right hand, behind the tree stump. Then she jerked up both hands and held a small cuddly toy in her right hand. The friends applauded, but a little hesitantly.

"Um ..." said the little hedgehog, "Did you get the stuffed animal out of the cylinder? Or behind the tree stump, conjured up? "" Well, tell me! "The small field mouse was awakened. "Out of the cylinder, of course!" She asserted. "That looked different," confirmed the little frog. "Yes, exactly!" The little hedgehog again invaded. "Somehow, your 'magic' does not seem quite professional." The small field mouse lowered its head. "Yes, you are right. Actually, I can not do magic. "" Shall I teach you? "Asked the little pink piggy.

64

"You want to teach me magic?" Wondered the little field mouse. "Can you do that anyway?" "Klaro!" Came in response and a surprised murmur made the rounds among friends. "Show us!" Demanded the little hedgehog, who could not believe that. And the little piglet exchanged the position with the little field mouse. "Ladies and Gentlemen," it began, "now watch the famous and infamous magic show of the little pink pig!" Behavioral clapping began. The friends were not sure yet what to expect now.

"First," the magician continued, "I'll let this cuddly toy" the cuddly toy was shaken in the hand, "disappear in the cylinder!" Until now, the show did not look so bad and the little field mouse drummed with their paws a kind of drum roll on the tree trunk. The little pink piggy put the stuffed animal in the cylinder and covered it with the cloth. "Hocus and pox, the cuddly toy now disappears, but not only to the locus, but in every sense of the wind!" It waved mystically with his arms over the cylinder and pulled the cloth abruptly aside. "Ta-Taaaa!" Shouted it, putting itself in victory pose.

"Huh?" The little hedgehog let out. "The cuddly toy is still in the cylinder." "Nonsense, is not it!" Replied the pig and lifted the cylinder up and turned it around loosely Gaaaanz. When the cuddly toy should have fallen out, it did not happen. The friends got big eyes. "Where is it?" Wondered the little frog and hopped forward and examined the cylinder. In the cylinder was no cuddly toy. And there was no one behind the tree stump and the piggy had obviously no cuddly toy with him. "Hey!" Cried the little hedgehog, "you can actually do magic!" "I say!" Insisted the little pink pig.

"Then you can really teach me?" Asked the little field mouse. "Klaro!" But before that the magic show continued. "Ladies and gentlemen! Watch me spell out the cuddly toy again! "The small field mouse again made its drum roll on the tree trunk. The little frog looked at the piggy with big eyes. There's a catch, he thought, the pig CAN NOT conjure. "Aboro co Diboro! Singa Pur and Qudra Tur! Cuddly toy now come out, preferably here and not in the moor. "And again, the little piggy

65

wagged over the cylinder with the cloth on it. "TA-TAAAA!" Cried it, tore its arms up again and made the winning pose.

The clapping was a bit louder now but stopped quickly. "I do not see it yet," the little frog grumbled again. "Should that be in the cylinder now, or what?" "Ladies and gentlemen, I'm going to turn this cylinder around slowly now." And the piggy turned the cylinder gaaaanz loosely as before. And again, no cuddly toy fell out. "The cuddly toy is NOT in the cylinder. Where can it be? I've conjured it up again. "" Come on, you bang bag, tell me! "Cried the frog, who still thought it all a big scam. "My dear frog, please turn around once," said the little pink piggy.

The frog turned and saw the cuddly toy sitting on its feet behind the tree trunk on which they sat. It seemed to be smirking at the little frog. He took the cuddly toy amazed and held it up for everyone to see. And again, the pig called, "TA-TAAAAAAA!" But now the friends were clapping wildly and loud and loud. "Bravo!" "Great!" "Great!" Shouted the three spectators and the little frog patted the piggy's shoulder. "You can REALLY conjure!" And the little hedgehog rejoiced: "I know a magician! I know a magician! "

In the next few days, the little field mouse learned magic from the little pink piggy. It was not easy. It took a lot of effort to get the difficult exercises done. Some magic tricks went pretty easy. But others were really hard to learn. After a few days, she showed her friends some tricks. The friends were really excited about how well she had learned magic. They clapped, cheered and shouted for encore. At the encore, the little pink piggy had to help out a bit. But that was the best magic show the friends had ever seen and organized.

CHAPTER 13

The Custodian

I was born Oxford Aaron Jacobson on October 7th. 2018 in San
Diego, California, to James Wilson Jacobson and Janine Anne
Jacobson. Both of my parents were clairvoyant, as were both of
their respective parents. I have "gifts" beyond those ever known in the
modern history of the Earth. Some have called me a superhero because
I help those in need and fight against oppression and hunger. Some have
called me a savior because I speak in the xenoglossia and work with
augury. I am, however, a mere mortal and desire no special treatment
from any man.

When I was a newborn, I saw the trees swaying outside my nursery
window and pointed to them when my parents were near. They
understood and made a safe area for me to experience the natural
surroundings of the outdoors. I loved the way the trees moved when
the wind lightly fluttered through their branches. I marveled at the
clouds and the non-linear formations and fractals that they endlessly
created. I listened to the audible sounds of birds, insects, and other
animals and understood what they were saying. I absolutely loved the
colors of the planet that were everywhere in nature and the never-ending
spiral curves of each component of it all. Non-geometric patterns, I
noted, ruled growth and the manifestation of life.

When I was 4 years of age, my parents brought to me a whiteboard and
a chalkboard. They knew I would deliver arcane information. They
wanted to know if I would choose the chalk or the dry erase pens. Both
had placed their faith on the chalkboard, and that is the one I chose. On
that chalkboard, I wrote the definitions of words that were never

spoken. I set about the creation of machines to help the world operate on a cleaner and more efficient scale. I defined equations that led to the design and eventual manufacture of means of transportation and defense that revolutionized a great deal of what we see today, and I gave chemists, scientists, and surgeons, answers to how to prevent and illuminate physical conditions and detriments that, if left unanswered, would have caused mass pain and death in society's all around the globe.

When I was 10, the local police and detectives asked for my help with their work.

This I did to some degree but quickly learned that it was below my station and, after making accurate assessments of the problems and the nature of the issues they faced, I quickly located, trained and accredited other qualified individuals and instrumentally placed them in positions with the local and state police, as well as the FBI and in some cases, the government. After doing this, I placed myself into globally leaning endeavors in helping those in foreign lands who had been cut off from civil surroundings, and whose habitat had become severely compromised. Those were the victims of the power-hungry and the greedy who would use the backs of others to climb to temporary, pseudo heights. It is true that I do fight evil.

Today, I am the CEO of a multi-national corporation that creates software and equipment for large companies that build computing platforms and space systems. At least that is what the government believes. My venerate persona is crucially challenged by this deceit, and only the power of my mental armor protects me from the influence of guilt and shame in the name of honor among men of decree.

There are no insiders in my firm, only those who I hold dear, and their family members, understand what my intentions truly are. There are no visitors to the areas in my buildings which house the real workings of my business. It is a front. We do hire good normal people to create software, and we do make a profit from doing so, but all that is only a ruse to allow me to do what I do best. Help those who need help and those who cannot help themselves.

We make replicators and carry them to countries like Africa and farm equipment that produce accelerated growth crops inside of a week for those who have access to land but are repressed from otherwise doing so. Our labs are exclusive to this planet. We manufacture nanomachines that can build anything and do anything.

One top-secret area creates what we like to call peace machines. These are nanobots that slowly inhibit the bloodstream of those oligarchs who would serve only the health of themselves by trampling the rights and needs of others. They never know why they begin to get sick and slowly die, they just do, and then we go in and eliminate any remnants of their filthy existence so no history can ever know of their hatred and fears. These nanos are used with extreme care, and only when selected individuals are deemed impossible to rehabilitate. In that situation, only one platform is available. Regretfully, this is unanimous in its determination and its results.

My team personally travels with all the equipment in question and teaches the suffering masses how to operate these tools in a clandestine manner. In this way, we are making strong communities in areas of the world generally dominated by greedy pea-brained thugs who love only power, money, and violence.

We also make a series of covert products that work by utilizing nanotechnology for medical purposes. Our technology has the power to easily re-grow limbs and internal organs, and also regeneration beds that enable life extension. We apply these services, beginning at the bottom and moving up from there. The poor and homeless, the downtrodden and weak, always get what they need immediately. We are here to make lives better and push the evil global powers onto the ash heaps of history.

There is also one other piece of very valid and exclusive technology that we alone build that we do not sell or reveal to anyone else, and that falls into the area of time travel. When a tyrant shows up, and a timeline is initiated, we use our time tech to go back and prevent that tyrant from ever existing.

Now, I personally designed and assisted in the creation of something that could be called a weapon of peace. Before I explain what it is and how we use it, I must tell you why we made it. Often times, in the work we do in various places around the globe, a person or group of people make plans or begin an agenda that, through some of our other technologies, we know will lead to the death or poisoning of a great many innocent people, sometimes a large portion of an entire culture in societies. The prime directive covering what we do and what I stand for does not and cannot allow these types of events to happen, so we neutralize them long before they can come to fruition. This brings us back to the way in which we do it.

It is called an Adapter Beam Machine. It looks like a very small chromium tube and can easily be an integral part of a soldier's gear. It can also be carried in one's pocket. It is that small! The beam unit is so incredibly powerful that only those with an extreme degree of psionics are even allowed to handle it, and those same individuals are exclusively qualified to carry and utilize it. The beam is activated with a sequence of mental acuity and memory and requires a system of codes.

When we are on a mission and intend to use the Adapter Beam, the codes are already inserted by the mission specialist who carries it, and it is ready to fire.

Generally, this unit is utilized in conjunction with time travel adjustment missions. First, we track the progress of something negative that happened. We determine the answer to the question, "What happened?" Then, we follow the timeline taking into consideration all the people whom that timeline touches, and we track it all the way back to its inception. In this way, instead of having to remove or neutralize an entire league of politicians, soldiers, or criminals, we only need to focus on one. Without the initial idea, the dominoes never fall!

In essence, what this amounts to, is prevention. Prevent the conception of the kernel of an idea from ever coming into manifestation, and you have prevented the negative results that the idea would have spawned.

In the end, here is how that looks. We learn that a certain devious and violent group is planning to overthrow a government that is working, which is a peaceful and productive institution. Then, we go back in time and use the Adapter Beam to discharge the individual who is responsible for the inception of that agenda, and we have removed the problem before it ever begins, thereby saving thousands, sometimes millions of lives. We think that is a good idea and a great service to the planet.

How is it that the Adapter Beam is the one technology that alone can do this? When the Adapter is discharged, there is a very powerful blue beam; call this a laser beam if you like, although technically, this would be incorrect. The beam enters the receiver's brain and de-develops the brain patterns giving them the mentality of a 10-year-old. They are not damaged or hurt in any way, but rather simply rendered ineffective. The carrier of the Adapter Beam weapon never goes into a mission alone, because after the shot, the receiver needs immediate attention. They become disoriented as the new brain patterns begin to send out sensory data, and, in some cases, the recipient may even need actual support, so they don't fall over and hurt themselves. My men are there in an instant!

We bring this individual back with us and check them into special handling houses we have set up in various areas just for this purpose. In the course of a few months, they are placed back into society as janitors or night watchmen, something that requires little intelligence but provides a good degree of achievement on the part of the individual, while being totally innocuous in its essence. They are safe and well cared for during and after the entire ordeal. This is why the Adapter Beam Weapon is more a weapon of peace. The annihilation of a great many good law-abiding members of society is prevented, and a very bad

71

person is rendered good, and can never ever have those negative thought patterns again for as long as they shall live.

I am the custodian!

The End

CHAPTER 14

Story of the Little Annika

I tell you the story of little Annika ...

Annika pulls her blanket up to her chin, presses her teddy tightly to her and pinches her eyes. It does not help anything. She escapes night after night to her parents' safe nest. I can understand Annika very well.

What would you say as a parent so that she is not afraid anymore? Would you try to explain to her that there are no ghosts? Annika would protest. They exist very well! She can hear her. Yes, even feel it.

Annika's mother has an idea.

She places a small, green-shining moon in the nursery and tells her daughter, "Did you know that ghosts are afraid of green light?" Annika looks at her mother with wide eyes. "Ghosts are afraid too?" She asks. "Yes, and they can not harm you when the green moon shines for you."

Annika nods and understands.

Every time Annika hears another giggle or flashes and storms outside, she looks at the moon. She believes in him. Imagines that his green light envelops her. Trust in the wisdom and love of her mother and close her eyes calmly.

However, the story continues ...

Annika is growing up. At some point, she no longer needs the green light. The idea of witches and monsters is now funny.

However, completely different spirits appear in Annika's life.

The worry of not finding the right one. The concern that the money for the rent increase is not enough. The fear that she will never fit in her favorite jeans again ...

Do you think these ghosts are familiar?

Even thirty years later, she can not sleep again because of ghosts. She turns back to her mother.

"You know mom, I sometimes wallow in bed for hours. The worries just do not want to go away. "

"My little one, can you still remember the green moon that drove away all your spirits?"

"Yes. What do you mean by that? A plastic light will hardly be the solution to my worries. These are real! "

The mother laughed heartily.

"Worries are like ghosts. If you do not believe in them, they can not hurt you. Because worries or fears have only one power: they keep you from concentrating on what you want.

Your attention is like the headlight of a lighthouse. If he rests on what you want, he can not be with your worries. "

The mother chuckles happily and wants to get up. Everything is said for her.

You can not fight worries

"But mom, if I do not solve my worries, then stay! I have to think about her. "

"Have we been dealing with your spirits before? Has your closet broken down, trimmed the feet of your crib or called the Ghostbuster?

74

No, we did not fight your spirits because they do not exist. Only your attention has given them life. Likewise, your worries only exist in your head. If you try to solve or fight them, they stay alive. "

Annika reflects on her mother's words. If a stranger had told her that, she would have labeled him a reality refugee. However, she has watched her mother too many times, keeping her smile in any challenge. She never had the feeling that she was covering something.

Only now, after she herself knows the wrong ways and ups and downs of life, she appreciates this even more on her mother.

"OK," Annika says. "I'll give it a try. But I no longer believe in the protection of the green moon. I'm sorry."

The mother answers. "You have something much, much better. It's your wishes and dreams. Focus your spotlight on the places you see, the people you laugh with and the successes you want to celebrate.

I promise you that these pictures will come alive every day. "

We are faced with choices countless times every day, either directing our attention to our concerns or to our dreams.

Our life will be guided by this decision.

75

CHAPTER 15

Ali Mama and Her Forty Daughters

Ali Mama was already an old woman, worried about how they could survive in the desert.

How they got food, how to dress and feed her daughters, not a day went by that she wasn't worried. And despite the hot sun, she not only wrinkled because of it but mainly because of all the worries she had. She was already an old woman when her last daughter was born, and then she was only 60 years old. Ali Mama was once stolen from a harem, where the old salesman Marmar beheld her special Russian-Azarbaïdjan beauty and immediately concealed it and took it on his donkey to his desert village.

Ali Mama had given birth to forty daughters.

When she was 12 years old, she had to marry the old lusty man Marmar, who taught her all the tricks of the game of love, which of course, was never the case.

Ali Mama had never asked for that smelly bearded horny goat in her night's sleep.

He soon died because he was very old and possessed too much lust, leaving behind his young Ali Mama after one of the violent sexual tricks he had once learned in India. Now then, you knew it, upside down, behind, now a whole hassle, and he was finally suffocated, while Ali Mama leaned over his old weathered bearded goat beard.

Now Ali Mama was a very innocent and sweet girl at the time, and she did not know better whether he had died of natural death.

No one in the desert thought about it, and you shouldn't do that either, because it was way too hot for that.

But the old horny goat Marmar left his Ali Mama a house with 5 bedrooms and a large living room, a utility room and a hall, a goatee, a skinny bald cow, 2 chickens, and a donkey with a cart.

All in all, quite a lot for a desert resident who had become a merchant, even though he had traveled all over the world.

And Ali Mama stayed behind with her two little daughters and no one who wanted to look after her and her children.

Ali Mama, of course, also had to eat, and that is why the shutters and the back door opened wide at night.

Soon many men came to visit Ali Mama, and she taught them the game of love as she had learned from her former husband.

Now Ali Mama was enormously fertile, and God just poured his children over her fields.

Ali Mama became the richest woman in the desert village and not a woman who dared to speak badly about her because then the men were so angry that they did not give up their daily wages to their wives and children.

Men were already the boss there anyway, so what did those women have to bring in?

Nothing, nothing at all, just a kitchen counter and a bare, dry back garden, where they could sometimes grow some vegetables with pain and effort.

Ali Mama grew into a real Mama, with a strong front and back, and the men were crazy about her. Of course, they paid her for the expenses for all the daughters that she gave birth to.

Yet that was never enough.

As voluptuous as Ali Mama was, her daughters had to have a proper marriage. But how did she get these beautiful daughters out if no one knew who their fathers were in that village?

Many boys wanted to marry the daughter of Ali Mama, but for the same money, they married their half-sister.

Look at a cousin that didn't sin yet, but a half-sister or brother who, no, no none of it! Nothing came of it.

What would Ali Mama have to come up with to give her daughters a good life?

Forty daughters, including some twins, beautiful, with black almond-shaped eyes, some even blue! With beautiful jet-black long hairs, some with curls, some so stylish that it did look like Chinese beauty, very beautiful girls that everyone would lick their fingers off. But nobody was allowed to touch it, hardly even looking at it.

Ali Mama was desperate, sometime the day she would go and who would take care of her beautiful daughters? The daughters were able to weave beautiful rugs, that was clear. No one could do that as well as her daughters. Ali Mama herself could not weave at all.

But the back door was always open, no matter how old she was, the men still knew where to find her.

But no one touched her daughters, she didn't have to be afraid of anything, many men were afraid even to touch the beautiful girls, for the same money, you had such incest, and that was strictly forbidden there in that desert village.

Ali Mama decided that she had to do something and so she decided on a big trip, on her way to Persia, to look for forty men for her forty daughters.

Thought so done, the men in the village were inconsolable, if Ali Mama would come back because they would miss her so much. Ali Mama smiled at them and said: If God wants it!

Just like in a caravan, the parade started, a long line of beautiful girls, one a little older than the first-born and the other.

But that didn't matter after all?

Finally, after many hot days in the desert, they arrived in Persia. Right at the border, there was a big surprise. There was a villager, Ali Baba, and his forty sons.

Now that worked out well.

Ali Mama knocked on the door of Ali Baba's house, and when he opened the door and saw all those women, tears filled his eyes.

Ai, ai .... he exclaimed, clapping his hands with joy.

Look here, Allah has answered our prayers.

Forty women for my forty sons.

Ali Mama said exactly then, forty men for my forty daughters.

Now Ali Baba was enormously rich, and he wanted to accept all daughters as his daughters-in-law, not one except.

It turned out to be a terribly long party, forty days and nights, and everyday marriage was concluded between a son of Ali Baba and a daughter of Ali Mama.

They all became very happy.

Ali Baba with Ali Mama, because they just fell in love with each other, after forty days and agree with them?

The men in the village in the desert remained unhappy, but who cared if you were rich and could live in Persia at the time?

It was way too hot for everyone there.

And they lived happily ever after.

CHAPTER 16

Daisy and the Butterfly

D aisy, the fairy, could hop across lily pads and climb up snake grass.

She could paint pictures of ladybugs and summersault across the grass.

She could even create small sculptures out of clay that she found by the side of the creek.

One thing Daisy could not do, though, was fly.

When Daisy was born, her wings were broken and so she could not use them.

As she grew older, her wings grew more mangled and twisted and it became even more obvious that she would never be able to fly like the other fairies.

While Daisy had great fun enjoying her life, she always wished that she could fly as the other fairies did.

Sometimes, she would sit by herself and feel sad that while everyone else was playing tag in the air, she was left on the ground, unable to play with the others.

Daisy's family felt sad that she could not play with her friends all the time, so they did their best to always keep her company and help her have a great time.

One day, Daisy was making a sculpture by the Creekside when a giant butterfly landed nearby.

Enchanted by the beauty of this butterfly, Daisy walked right up to it and started looking at its big beautiful wings.

Daisy was surprised by how still and kind the butterfly seemed as she gazed at its beauty.

Most times, if Daisy walked up to them, butterflies would simply fly away and leave her by herself, wondering about their beauty.

This butterfly, though, was different.

As Daisy gazed at it and walked closer and closer, the butterfly's wings stopped moving, and it seemed as though the butterfly was nodding its head at her.

Curious, Daisy walked closer.

The butterfly again nodded its head as if it was inviting Daisy to sit on its back.

Slowly, Daisy climbed up onto the butterfly and sat on its back, wrapping her arms and legs around its body for support.

Once she was on the butterfly, the butterfly took off flying!

Daisy was surprised: she had never been in flight before.

When she was just a baby, her mom and dad would often fly around with her on their backs, but as she got older, Daisy got too heavy for them to carry.

This was Daisy's first time flying since she was so small!

At first, Daisy was scared, so she clung tight to the butterfly and closed her eyes.

She could feel the rush of cool air blowing against her face as they flew all around the forest.

After a few moments, though, Daisy relaxed and realized how fun it was to be flying.

She opened her eyes and watched as the trees, frogs, and flowers of the forest all floated by while they flew around the forest by the creek.

First, the butterfly simply flew around as if she was playing in the sunlight and dancing in the breeze that swept across the forest.

Soon, though, the butterfly seemed as if she was on a mission.

She started by going to a beautiful meadow filled with wildflowers.

There, the butterfly landed on each one and began drinking in the sweet nectar from the plants.

Daisy watched, surprised at how impressive it was to watch such a beautiful creature enjoying a delicious treat from a flower.

When she was done drinking, the butterfly flew to another flower, and then another one.

All around, bees were floating from flower to flower, too.

Daisy could also see many of her friends playing a game of tag in the distance.

For once, she knew what it felt like to be up in the air with them, even if she was not playing tag with her friends.

Daisy hugged the butterfly tighter now because she was so thankful that the butterfly was giving her such a special treat.

After the butterfly drank nectar from the flowers, she left the meadow and went back to the creek.

There, the butterfly began to drink water from the creek.

As she did, Daisy could feel the butterfly's belly swelling with a delicious meal and drink from the forest.

When she was done drinking, the butterfly took Daisy on another trip.

This time, they went high into the trees and landed on a small twig at the end of a long branch.

There, the butterfly rested for several minutes, digesting her meal and taking in the warmth of the sun.

Daisy relaxed and nestled into the back of the butterfly, enjoying a sweet rest with her new flighted friend.

When their rest was done, the butterfly began to go on the move once more.

This time, the butterfly went to a different meadow where they came across many different butterflies.

Some looked like the butterfly Daisy was riding, whereas others looked completely different.

When they arrived, some of the butterflies moved from flower to flower, gathering nectar just like Daisy's butterfly had done earlier.

Others opted instead to snack on fruits that were growing on trees on the edge of the meadow.

This time, the butterfly went to the trees and started snacking on some of the fruit.

Curious, Daisy reached out and grabbed a handful of fruit and tried some herself.

The fruit tasted sweeter and yummier than the fruits that she and her family usually ate, which were fruits that were connected from lower to the ground.

Daisy knew she was lucky and that this was a special treat that she would remember forever.

When they were done eating the special fruit, the butterfly began to fly back toward the creek where Daisy had been making clay sculptures.

Daisy held tight as they swooped and swirled through the air, enjoying a playful ride on their way back. She was giggling the whole time.

They finally landed back at the creek and Daisy hopped off of the back of the butterfly and landed on the ground on her own two feet.

She thanked the butterfly and gave the butterfly a big hug around the neck and asked if she would please come to visit again one day.

The butterfly nodded and smiled before flying off into the distance.

Daisy watched the colors of the enchanting butterfly as the sunlight caught her wings and created a beautiful spectacle for Daisy to watch.

As she got further away, the butterfly turned back and winked at Daisy, as if to thank her for a wonderful day, too.

Daisy was so happy from her day in the sky that she left her clay sculpture so she could finish it another day.

Instead, she happily walked back to her home with her mom and her dad and sat down at the dinner table to eat a snack with her family.

When her parents asked her why she was so happy, Daisy told them about her experience with the butterfly and how she had taken a wonderful flight around the forest.

She told them about the nectar, and the drink from the stream, and the fruits in the sky.

Surprised, Daisy's parents looked at each other and wondered how such a magical thing could possibly happen.

They were happy for their daughter and for her opportunity to fly with the rest of the fairies.

When Daisy went to sleep that night, she dreamt about soaring through the sky and enjoying a delicious sky fruit.

She felt so lucky to meet such a wonderful friend who would help her have a chance to fly in the sky as the other fairies did.

And, the butterfly did return many times.

Each time she returned, she would take Daisy on a flight around the forest and show her the new flowers, sky fruits, and bushes growing around the forest.

Daisy would never again be stuck on the ground with her new friend looking out for her.

What a lucky fairy Daisy was!

CHAPTER 17

A Mythical Land

Heavens existed beyond the Earth. Not above the Earth as some beings believed. Not within the Earth, as others theorized. Heavens were both beyond the Earth and around the Earth. There was a sense of separation, but it was not a physical separation in the measure of heights and distances. In fact, it was quite the opposite. The separation of Heavens from the Earth was one that came from both within and without. Rather than heights and distances, the separation was measured in depths and vibrations.

This was a lesson that was difficult for a mortal to comprehend. Of course, some are able to reach the realization. Some grasped a shred of a Chaos Theory from the Core Universe. Most were led to the conclusion by a being from Heavens. One such mortal would be Angus of the First Men. There was also Raven of the First Women. Of course, there was the Great Chief Howlite of the First Men and the Great Chieftess Lilith of the First Women. These ones, these very peculiar mortals, were led by a being they call the Sacred Flame. Over time, they had begun to grasp onto the origin of the Sacred Flame. What it truly was.

The Ancestors of Great Chief Howlite of the First Men and Great Chief Lilith of the First Women were the Wandering Tribe. The Wandering Tribe first encountered the being known as the Sacred Flame as something else entirely. A formless, nonphysical entity they dubbed as the Voice. The First Men and First Women who left the Empire before it burned believed the Voice might be something supernatural but had no certainty. They considered the fact that it might be a being from

87

another earth. Maybe a distant star? Or even a signal sent out across the universe. But none of them realized the truth. The descendants of the First Men and First Women, who called themselves the First Men and First Women, expanded on the theory. Somehow, these humans got closer to the truth, but further.

The First Men and the First Women that led the Wandering Tribe believed the Voice was a God of some kind. A guardian, a guide, and a deliverer from horrors that lay beyond their awareness. They were right on many levels, of course. But not in the ways they thought. The god they believed the Voice was is something nonexistent in this dimension. A god to these early mortals remained something that was simply beyond their realm of comprehension. A man from the 355th century could travel to the past and project himself as a god to these folks. A true god would be something closer to the realm of the Celestial Being, the beings of Chaos and Order, or things of the like. Those that came from the infinite. That both were and were not.

The reality of the god of the Wander Tribe, this Voice, later to be named the Sacred Flame, was much more tangible. In fact, Great Chief Howlite of the First Men and Great Chieftess Lilith of the First Women stepped foot upon the very tangible realm of origin for the Sacred Flame. It was during their brief visit to the cottage of Angus of the First Men and Raven of the First Women. Angus and Raven simply referred to the place as the "Spirit Realm," but it was much more than that. It was the place that most beings referred to as "Gods" had come from in this dimension. Spirits, deities, gods and goddesses, monsters and horrors, fairies and blessings, even the miracles the mortals might pray for. All of these things slipped from this "Spirit Realm," which would be better described as Heaven of this universe. In this place we will call Heaven, there were many beings like the Sacred Flame. Though not all of them were nearly as powerful. This is the story of the Sacred Flame and how it found itself trapped on the plane of the Earth and banished from Heaven.

The Sacred Flame had a far older and far more powerful name than "Sacred Flame," which would be unknown to humans of course. The Great Chief Howlite of the First Men and the Great Chieftess Lilith of the First Women did learn this name however, after learning the tongue that the beings of Heaven speak. It was an old language, and that made the name and the old one. And difficult to pronounce for young tongues. The True Name of the Sacred Flame was "Kyrxymvahlyrndrekkahlaerrenanodon". For the sake of everyone's sanity, we will refer to the Sacred Flame with a nickname. Let's go with Vahl. So, Vahl's origin in Heaven was dated back to a time before most of its denizens. She was one of the first beings to come to life on that dimensional frequency. Due to this, she was able to exist for longer, giving her more power when other beings came to life there. That is why she would be labeled as a "God" in the hierarchy of Heaven. The God was the oldest spirit known in Heaven, which even Vahl did not know. A god was one of the strongest and oldest spirits to exist Heaven. An angel was one of the more powerful spirits, but younger than a god. From there, it went spirit, nymph, sprite, pixie, wisp, and mote. As you can imagine, they digress in order of power and age.

So yes, Vahl was considered a god of Heaven. She was one of the oldest, wisest, and most powerful. However, she was not arrogant or cruel. In fact, her eons of existence what was once a hotheaded young spirit into a placid angel and a compassionate god. She did have ambition. Her dream was to become the God. Since she had never met one, she believed it never existed. But there was no rush for her to get there. For the time being, Vahl was content to coexist with the other gods and celebrate existence. There was the Golem of Crystal, Lione. He was a representation of discipline and perseverance. There was the Two-Headed Mountain Giantess Ghulu, the embodiment of patience and open-mindedness. And finally, there was the Sage Dragon Solomon, the epitome of wisdom and foresight. Together with Vahl, these four gods stood as the four oldest of the gods in Heaven.

To the younger spirits, this group was called the Four. The Four were responsible for maintaining balance and tranquility in the realms of Heaven and the Earth. Of them, Vahl was the oldest. She was the illumination of compassion and guidance. Her charge was to not only guide and oversee the other three of the Four but also to watch over every other angel, spirit, nymph, sprite, pixie, wisp and mote. Given the many she had to watch over, it understandable that Vahl had many eyes. In fact, upon her entire form of silver-blue fire, which rose over one hundred feet high and wielded many limbs, Vahl watched with over one thousand eyes. Those one thousand eyes were responsible for watching over and protecting not just those spirits in Heaven, but the ones sent down to the Earth as well.

Vahl was beloved by most of the beings in the realms. Heavens sang her praises and the Earth thanked her for her vigilance in their protection. During her time as the Old God of the Four, not a soul went on persecuted. Not on the Earth and never in Heaven. But over eons of service and dedication, one can grow blind to those closest to them. It was the Sage Dragon, Solomon, that warned her of this first.

"Vahl. Often it is those closest to us that we can be the most blind to. And some may grow so close to you on purpose, so they may escape your sight. Be wary of the dangers that lurk near."

"Oh, Solomon. You are kind and generous to offer me your sage advice. But I vow to you; my eyes are never blind. I watch all without yielding." Vahl shimmered in the infinite light that populated Heaven. Her flames danced as she burned with mirth.

Why? Why would the oldest god of the gods not heed the words of the wisest god, the god who quite literally embodied wisdom? Solomon was Vahl's oldest friend. But Vahl was complacent.

She had grown accustomed to all being wary of her ire that she did not realize some had grown foolish in several eons of compassion. Once Vahl was feared as a god. The fires she could rain upon a spirit would send them banished the most painful ways. But even the memories of ancient beings were not so long as it should.

In the end, Solomon was right. There was a plot against her. Ghulu, the Two-Headed Mountain Giantess, had raised a plot to knock Vahl down so she could wake her way up. Ghulu, without another soul knowing, had befriended the God. Little to her surprise, it was a mild and unassuming spirit. In the form of a simple cloud, it went along through Heaven and watched all. But Ghulu, in all her evil ways, gained the trust of the God only to kill it. She planned to pin the deed on Vahl, labeling her as a power-hungry god who would do anything to be the God. And unfortunately for Vahl, Ghulu's plan mostly worked. Ghulu did kill the God, as much as the God can be killed. In its final acts before reincarnation, the God spent its energy to cast two judgments.

The first judgment was cast on Ghulu. Ghulu was branded a God Killer. This was the worst title a spirit could ever be given. With this brand, never could a spirit enter Heaven again. But to ensure that remained so, the God shattered Ghulu. He tore her apart into a thousand monstrosities. Horrific, frog-like creatures with long and disjointed arms that wield two grotesque claws. Her back was adorned with a hardened shall and her tongue was replaced with lashing tentacles. Split into a thousand of these horrors, forever called Ghouls; the God Killer was banished to the Earth. But Ghulu was not the only one to suffer. For failing as the oldest of the gods, Watcher of Heaven and the Earth, Vahl was banished to the Earth as well. The God reduced Vahl to a wisp, just one step above mote. He sentenced her to a penance there that would last eons. On the Earth, Vahl must be more vigilant than ever before. With no power and no eyes, she must learn how to protect the Earth and all its inhabitants. She must earn the title Watcher of the Earth before she may again earn the title Watcher of Heaven.

Now that you know why Vahl was sent to the Earth, transformed into the Sacred Flame, what she has done may make more sense to you. Vahl works constantly to atone her failure. To make up for not protecting the God and her fellow spirits, the Sacred Flame aims to become the

91

Protector of the Earth. She will not rest until the days she does so. And without the power of her own, she has learned to world closely and through the humans who are worth it. Such as the Great Chief Howlite of the First Men and the Great Chieftess Lilith of the First Women. She will protect the world with all her spirit. She will never rest.

CHAPTER 18

After the Fair

The fair was already closed, the lights on the stalls where they sold the coconut slices had been turned off, and the little wooden horses, motionless in the dark, awaited the music and the run of the machinery that would set them jogging again. In the booths, the mothballs had gone out one by one, and the canvases covered the game boards one by one. The entire crowd had returned home, and there was only a little light left in the caravan windows.

No one had noticed that girl. Leaning on the side of the roundabout, dressed in black completely, I heard the last rumor of the already distant steps that were marked on the sawdust and the murmur of goodbyes. Then, alone in the middle of that desert of horses of profile and humble fantastic boats, he began to look for a place to spend the night. Here and there, raising the canvases that covered the stalls as if they were shrouds, it made its way into the darkness. He was scared of mice running around junk-filled entablements, and he was afraid of the same fluttering of the canvas that the air wobbled like the sails of a ship. He had hidden by the merry-go-round. It slipped inside, and with the creaking of the steps the bells that the horses had hung around their neck rang. He dared not breathe until the quiet silence resumed and the darkness had not forgotten the noise. In all the gondolas, in all the positions I looked with my eyes for a bed to lie on, but there was not a single place in the whole fair where I could go to sleep. Some because they were too quiet, others because of the mice. In the astrologer's post was a pile of straw. He knelt on his side and when he reached out he felt that he was touching a child's hand. In the astrologer's post was a pile of straw. He knelt on his side and when he reached out he felt that he was touching a child's hand. In the astrologer's post was a pile of straw. He knelt on his side and when he reached out he felt that he was touching a child's hand.

No, there wasn't a single place. Slowly, he went to the wagons that were farther from the center of the fair and discovered that there were lights in only two of them. He held his empty bag tightly and remained undecided while deciding which one he was going to bother. Finally, he chose to knock on the window of a small and decrepit one that was there next door. On tiptoe, he looked inside. In front of a kitchenette, toasting a slice of bread, sat the fattest man I had ever seen. He tapped three knuckles on the glass and then hid in the shadows. He heard the man go up the steps and ask: "Who? Who?". But he dared not answer. "Who? Who?" He repeated.

The man's voice, as thin as thick was his body, made him laugh.

And he, upon discovering the laughter, turned to where the darkness hid it.

"First call," he said, "then you hide and then laugh, huh?"

The girl then appeared in a circle of light, knowing that she no longer needed to remain hidden.

"A girl," said the man. Go on, get in and shake your feet.

He didn't even wait for her; He had already retired inside the wagon, and she had no choice but to follow him, climb the steps and get into that messy knife. The man had sat down again and was still toasting the same slice of bread.

-Are you there? He asked, because at that moment he turned his back.

-I close the door? Asked the girl. And he closed it without waiting for an answer.

He sat on a cot and watched him toast the bread.

94

"I know how to toast bread better than you," said the girl.

"I have no doubt," said the Fat man.

He saw that he placed a piece of charred bread on a plate and saw that he immediately put another in front of the fire. It burned immediately.

"Let me toast it," she said. And he clumsily extended the fork and the entire bar.

"Cut it," he said, "take it and eat it."

She sat in the chair.

"Look how you have sunk my bed," said the Fat man, "who are you to sink my bed?"

"My name is Annie," he said.

He immediately had all the toast and buttered bread, and the girl arranged it on two plates and brought two chairs to the table.

"I'm going to eat mine in bed," said the Fat man. Take it here.

When they finished dinner, he pushed his chair away and began to contemplate it from the other end of the table.

"I am the Fat," he said. I'm from Treorchy The fortune teller next door is from Aberdare.

"I'm not from the fair," said the girl. I come from Cardiff.

"Cardiff is a very big city," the Fat man nodded. And asked him why he was there.

"For money," Annie said.

And then he told him things about the fair, the places he had walked, the people he had met. He told him how old he was, what he thought, what his brothers were called and how he would like to put his son. He showed him a postcard of the port of Boston and a portrait of his mother, who was a weightlifter. And he told her what summer was like in Ireland.

"I've always been that fat," he said, "and now I'm already Fat." Because I'm so fat, nobody wants to touch me.

He talked about a heat wave in Sicily, he talked about the Mediterranean. She told him about the boy he had found in the astrologer's position.

"That's because of the stars again," he said.

"That child is going to die," Annie said.

He opened the door and went out into darkness. She did not move. He looked around, thinking that maybe he had gone to look for a policeman. It would be a fatality to be caught again by the police. On the other side of the open door, the night was inhospitable, and she brought the chair to the kitchen.

"If you are going to catch me, you better get caught hot," he told himself.

From the noise, he knew that the Fat man was approaching and began to tremble. He climbed the steps like a mountain with legs, and she clenched her hands under her skinny chest. Despite the darkness, he saw that the Fat man was smiling.

"Look what the stars have done," he said. He had the astrologer's boy in his arms.

She cradled him. The boy whined in his lap until he was silent. The girl told her the fear that had happened after she left.

"What would I do with a cop?"

She told him that a policeman was looking for her.

"And what have you done to get you looking for the police?"

96

She did not answer. Only the child was taken to the sterile chest. And he saw how thin she was.

"You have to eat, Cardiff," he said.

And then the boy began to cry. With a groan, the crying began to turn into a storm of despair. The girl rocked it, but nothing could relieve it.

-Shut up, shut up! Said the Fat, but the crying was still increasing. Annie suffocated him with kisses and caresses, but the screams persisted.

"We have to do something," she said.

"Sing her a babysitter."

He did so, but the boy did not like it.

"We can only do one thing," he said. We have to take it to the merry-go-round.

And with the boy hugged around his neck, he hurried down the carriage stairs and ran through the fair, deserted, while the Fat man was panting at his heels.

Between stalls and stalls they reached the center of the fair, where the roundabouts were, and climbed into one of the mounts.

"Start it," she said.

From a distance the Fat man could be heard circling the handlebar with which the mechanism that put the horses to gallop the entire day began to run. She heard the jerky run of machinery well. At the foot of the horses, the boards shuddered in a crunch. The girl saw that El Gordo leveraged a crank and saw him sit on the saddle of the smaller horse. The merry-go-round began to spin slowly at first, but quickly gained speed. The boy who was carrying the little girl now didn't cry anymore: he was beating his palms. The air of the night curled his hair, music vibrated in his ears. The little horses kept going around and round, and the trembling of their hooves silenced the wails of the night wind.

And that's how the people of the fair began to come out of their wagons, and thus they found the Fat man and the girl in black who carried a little boy in his arms. In their mechanical steeds they circled and more laps, to the beat of an organ music that was increasing.

CHAPTER 19

Autumn dreams

Jenny shook her head in dismay as she looked at her child, sitting amid a veritable pile of candy wrappers.

A cold Autumn breeze rolled in through the window and she got up to shut it.

"What am I going to do with you, kiddo? You are going to be up all night, bouncing off the walls with all that sugar! What was I thinking?"

Kirsty literally bounced on the bed, her gap-toothed grin fueled by entirely too much chocolate and marshmallow.

"Best Halloween ever, Mommy! I got, like, a hundred pounds of candy!"

Jenny laughed. The girl's enthusiasm was, if nothing else, infectious.

"I don't think quite that much, sweetie, but if you did, I'd box most of it up for next year!"

"Ewww!" Kirsty wrinkled her nose. "I don't want to eat year-old candy!"

"I didn't say you'd have to eat it!" laughed Jenny.

"Maybe we'll give it to your father as punishment for letting you eat so much candy tonight!"

She sighed. Sometimes that man just did not think about things before jumping into them, and Jenny was left cleaning up the mess.

Kirsty giggled uncontrollably. "I bet he'd barf!"

"I'm sure."

"Do you think he would barf so much it'd fill up my candy bag, Mama?"

"Oh, gross, young lady! Let's not talk about such things before bed!"

Jenny reached out and lightly touched the tip of Kirsty's nose with her finger.

"Now, how am I ever going to get you to sleep in this condition? It's an impossible task!"

"What about a story, Mommy?"

Jenny put a finger to her lips and paused in thought.

"You know what? That's not a bad idea!"

She went to the self and picked up a well-worn paperback.

"No, not that one!"

Jenny's fingers glided over to a thin storybook.

"Nope! The big one!"

Jenny picked up the heavy book with the crackling cover.

"Yes!"

As she sat on her daughter's bed, Kirsty managed to bounce even higher in anticipation.

"This book is the best one, Mommy! The stories in it really come to life! Better than the other ones."

"Okay, this one it is, sweetie. Now lay your head back and let me find a good one."

Though its covers were weathered, as Jenny slowly turned the pages to find the right story, they felt glossy and new as when she herself was a kid.

"Let me see, let me see...."

One-chapter page stood out. A corridor of trees with leaves of red and gold arcing over a long road.

A lone branch had fallen in the road, a slender arm with a single thin shoot reaching away from the main branch.

It resembled a numeral "6," surrounded by falling leaves. As the mother and daughter watched, a few more leaves fluttered lightly to the ground.

"This is perfect for a brisk Autumn night. We have got a toasty fire going downstairs. If you listen, you can almost hear its warm crackle...."

Glimpses of a sunset through the trees sprawled red, orange, and purple across the Autumn sky.

The wind rustled the branches and fanned the leaves like crackling flames of red and gold that arced overhead.

Jaina felt as though she walked through a warm fire on the hearth itself.

The air was fresh but brisk with the Fall sweeping through, and alive with the energy of changing seasons.

She breathed in deeply and the air smelled of pumpkin patches, spiced apples, tree sap, and the wood fires burning.

This time of year, had a special resonance as Summer gave way to Winter and the changes that swept in before the leaves fell.

Nights like tonight were magic. A living dream.

She almost needed no sleep; to walk down the street on such a night was as invigorating as any night's rest.

As Halloween approached, the world came to life with creatures and half-glimpsed spirits rarely seen outside of this time.

The change was upon the world, in the rich scents that wafted through the air of baking pies, of sweet apples upon the trees, of cold drafts from distant lands, and fires upon the hearth.

Smoke drifted from the chimneys as she passed rows of houses. Orange light shone warmly in the windows against the darkening world. The faded blue scarf she kept wrapped around her neck trailed behind her in the breeze.

There was a field at the end of the street that Jaina had loved since she was a child. It was fenced off now; full of tall grass, and the derelict structures she had played with was long gone.

An old rusted tractor. Concrete chunks left from a house demolished long ago. A small hill with an old well.

She had made up so many stories about the lives that went unfolded in that place, the staging site for her adventures into distant castles and faraway lands, or lazy summer naps with her friends while the butterflies flitted slowly overhead.

In Autumn, though, with a scarf around her neck and the change of seasons thick in the air, that field would serve as the gateway to many tales. As the butterflies changed through chrysalis, as the land changed during the Autumn, so did her stories involve metamorphosis.

Jaina walked through the gap in the fence, her fingertips trailing over the cold metal links.

A shiver ran through her as she crossed the threshold, but not because of the cold metal's touch; because she had stepped across the gateway and into another world.

The grass rose up around her steps, rippling in a sudden wind. Lights like fireflies appeared above trails that formed in the grass as hidden things scurried away.

A breath of wind spiraled around her, carrying with it leaves and memory: nutmeg and spice, a steaming hot cup of cocoa in the hands, smoke from the hearth fires, a soft but warm glow as the family huddled around the fireplace and shared stories. The perfect time of year.

Everything was transforming around her. Flowers opened in the field and then fell into slumber again.

Jaina knelt down, hearing a strange sort of symphony in the growth and decline of the flowers.

A hum, like an old playground song, or the music her mother would play as they all danced between kitchen and living room, preparing a celebratory feast as fiery-colored leaves carpeted the yard. And there!

Jaina turned and she saw an aged barrel sitting there in the grass amid a cloud of fireflies and butterflies. Water sloshed in the barrel and the smell of fresh apples filled the air.

The sound of laughter and children's voices followed, and then she saw them, as though they had just sprung from the tall grass.

One of the children was her. Some of them stood on stepstools made of logs. The older ones were tall enough to stand.

They took their turns bobbing for the apples, splashing each other with cold water, giggling like mad.

Leaves of yellow and red swirled about the outside of the scene, like a shifting wall between dream and waking worlds.

Jaina smiled, seeing her older sister push her head into the water before she was ready.

Young Jaina came up sputtering, a leaf sticking in her matted hair. She had been so furious with Melanie that day!

Looking back at it, she laughed. What she would give to go back to that time when her biggest worry was her siblings tormenting her!

Turning to her right, Jaina saw another wall of leaves before her, which parted as she approached.

This time she stepped into a scene she remembered all too well: the night of her thirteenth birthday party.

Jaina's whole family had gathered in the front room with Grandma Gail; that was the last birthday she would ever spend with her grandma.

The old woman smiled at her over her glasses, saving the best present for last. Jaina remembered it well: the very scarf she wore around her neck.

Grandma had knitted it herself over weeks, in Jaina's favorite color: a cool blue, like the Springtime morning sky.

She touched the fabric with her fingertips, still as soft as ever. Some of the colors had faded over ten years, but none of its comfort or warmth.

Grandma Gail had made it especially for those cooler Autumn nights that Jaina loved to explore.

Gail looked up and met Jaina's gaze with her kindly smile. Jaina's heart leaped. A breath caught in her throat.

She stood transfixed as Grandma Gail raised a hand and waved to her.

Of all sitting in the living room, only young Jaina noticed, and she turned her head, searching for whatever her dear grandmother saw.

Young Jaina shrugged and turned back to her scarf, holding it up in the firelight. She wrapped it around her neck and beamed a smile as Gail turned back to her.

104

Both of their eyes lit up as they shared a special moment that would make one of Jaina's favorite memories.

The leaves shifted again and Jaina found herself walking beside a creek in a forest. Late afternoon sunlight shone through a golden-red canopy.

She remembered the area well: she had walked here often as a child, and later would bring the young man who would one day become her husband on their first tentative date.

This time she was walking behind herself, as a young Jaina balanced precariously walking along a log fallen across the creek.

Older Jaina smiled, knowing what was coming. "Watch your step!" she called, and it seemed like her younger counterpart heard something through the mists of dream and memory.

She paused, but it was too late. Her foot slipped on moss and she tumbled into the creek with a splash.

The water was bitter cold. Jaina came up spluttering and gasping for air, shocked by the frigid water. She laughed and clambered out onto the shore.

Of course, she had to go back to dry off next to a fire in the backyard, but first, she saw what had caused her to slip: a small cocoon hanging on the knot where she was about to put her foot.

She had noticed it at the last second and trying to avoid it threw off her balance.

Young Jaina found that the timing was more blessed than cursed, however: the chrysalis was beginning to hatch.

A butterfly with drooping wings slowly crawled its way out of the cocoon, taking its first tentative steps as a young adult into an unsure world.

Jaina brushed dripping wet locks of hair from her eyes as she watched, shivering but fascinated.

The butterfly's wings slowly spread as it dried in the brisk Autumn air, patterned blue upon white, trimmed with black. A first few uncertain flaps tested the air.

Both Jainas watched with a bittersweet smile; both faced similar uncertainties, her younger self rapidly growing to meet the greater challenges of the world, and her older self-having struggled with those challenges.

Even now, she had to work hard and fight to make her own place in the world.

Yet here, in the dreams of Autumn, those burdens were laid aside. For like the butterfly, as it spread its wings with vigor and took to the sky, she had undergone her own metamorphosis.

From a girl to a young woman who had made her family proud, Jaina had learned to fly on her own as well.

She watched the butterfly as it fluttered up and around her, rising into the shafts of sunlight filtering down through the leaves. A trail of sparkling dust floated behind it like a river of tiny stars.

Jaina reached up and passed her hand through it, and when she drew it back, it seemed like she held for a moment a glimpse of the entire universe shining. Growth. Transition. Metamorphosis.

As the butterfly had undergone its many challenges to become who it was meant to be, so was she undergoing her own changes.

106

Smiling, the older Jaina turned away. She remembered falling into the creek, but until now had forgotten what made her slip.

Now she felt that it was worth the cold and the discomfort to witness something so beautiful.

Her own thoughts rose with the wind like a fluttering leaf, whispering through the trees and into a starry evening sky.

Below her, the forest unfolded like a vast meadow of apple-red and sunshine-gold.

Ribbons wound through it in the form of the streams and creeks, helping to shape a vast tapestry.

The leaves would fall and carpet the ground in royal beauty, and the trees would stand naked in their beauty for a season.

Seeds slept in the earth's firm embrace, buds dreamed upon the branches. A blanket of frost covered all, turning to glisten dew in the morning sun.

Through it, all the land and all its dreaming creatures continued to grow and transform to find their Spring. For now, in Autumn's sweet embrace, the world slept and Jaina floated above it in peaceful memory.

CHAPTER 20

A Tropical Island

Will you tell me more about the dolphins, Mommy?"

"Finish brushing your teeth first!" Jenny called into the bathroom.

The silly child poked her head out of the bathroom, toothbrush in hand, lips covered in toothpaste.

"Okie, Mom!" Flecks of toothpaste flew as she said it, and then grinned with foamy teeth.

Kirsty came out wiping her mouth with the back of her long sleeve and hopped into the bed as Jenny pulled back the covers.

"I really like the dolphins, Mom. They know how to have fun!"

"They do." Jenny nodded. "But there are all kinds of dreams to explore, you know. There is an entire world full of them out there. All kinds of perspectives you never imagined."

"What does 'perspective' mean, Mommy?"

Jenny tapped a finger to her lips. "It's…it's a way you view the world. Do you know how you got to see the forest dreaming from the fox's view? That's a new perspective."

"Oh, okay! So, what kind of per-spec-tive are we going to see tonight?"

Jenny opened the book; it is cover crackling. She flipped through the pages until she came to the next chapter.

"Oh, yes. This is a special one."

She turned the book so that Kirsty could properly see the picture.

It depicted a tropical island, thick with palm trees and ferns, and fallen coconuts on the beach forming a pattern that looked like the numeral "3."

Above it, in the swaying branches and green canopy, peeked all sorts of brightly colored birds.

Their many calls mingled with the sound of the lapping waves to create a light and hopeful background.

The scent of salt and the pungent fragrance of tropical plants drifted from the pages.

"Now, sweetie, let me show you what the dolphins were so keen to get to explore, but from a different perspective…."

Jaina woke up on a beach, but not the beach she had left.

Now instead of a sandy path back to the city, she found herself on a tropical island.

Coconuts littered the sand at her feet.

Bright red and spiky fruits hung in some of the trees.

A warm tropical wind blew past, stirring the leaves with a whispering rustle and billowing her hair.

Jaina smiled as she breathed it in. The air smelled so fresh, a lingering tang on her tongue.

She turned toward the nearby jungle.

A small bird with green feathers and a shiny blue around its head hopped down from one of the branches. "Welcome!" it chirped. "This is my home. Do you like it?"

109

Jaina nodded enthusiastically. "It's wonderful. So warm and cozy and peaceful. How do you ever stay awake here? I think I would spend my day napping if I lived in such a nice place!"

"Oh, but you don't know what else there is to see!" said Bird. "You would have no time for napping all day if you could see the beauty of this place!"

"Could I? Could you show me?" Jaina looked hopeful, her eyes big and bright. A bird could not resist her plea.

"Yes, I will show you. Come with me and see what only one on the wing can see! Then you tell me if you would spend all day napping."

"Deal!"

Jaina held out her arm, and Bird alighted upon it, tilting its head back and forth to stare at her with each eye.

"And…let the wind takes us!"

Then it flew off again, and Jaina found that she was looking at the beach from high above.

She was like Bird, winging her way through warm blue skies to appreciate the jungle and the ocean from on high.

She circled higher and higher, and the whole island became a green-carpeted seed below her.

Up until this high in the sky, only the winds kept her company, singing of the distant waves, of the past and the future.

"Here we go!" Bird dove down, tucking her wings, as the green jungle rushed up to meet her. She spread her wings and arced smoothly into level flight, circling the treetops.

Below her, she saw the coconuts sitting in the trees, humming softly in the breeze.

Harsh voices rose up to meet her: monkeys leaping from branch to branch, picking the fruits and eating them with lyrical delight.

They looked up at Bird as she flew past and waved their hands in envy.

Into the canopy, she plunged.

Green fan-shaped leaves fluttered in the wind as she flew past.

Other birds, some of them yellow with black beaks, and some of the dark blue with yellow beaks, and still others red with white markings sang loudly, all competing voices.

They looked up as she flew past. Some rose into the air with a flutter of feathers, but they could not keep up with her speed.

She wove through corridors of green and tan, leaves and branches adorned with fruits or coconuts, nimbly winging around tree trunks, dodging hanging vines, and great big spiderwebs glistening with morning dew like living chandeliers.

The chorus of chirps and hooting cries followed her as she raced through a blur of the jungle.

Then she was free and flew out over the beach, above the water.

Fish leaped and swam in the cerulean waves, all aglow from the sunshine warming the world.

Dolphins cavorted off the shore, leaping high from white-capped waves to glisten in the sun and crash back down again.

Bird Jaina watched the shadows darting about beneath the surface, and then she turned back to the island.

Flocks of seabirds circled on the shores, diving down to peck at some meal washed ashore.

"Food! Food! Food!" their cries said. The bird had more on her mind than simply eating.

111

She circled the island, white sand streaming by beneath her, the lush jungle rotating slowly in her eyes.

Slender fingers of sunlight crept through the canopy and golden dust swirled in their grasp.

Little lizards and dark beetles crawled up the trunks, racing to the top to reach the sunlight. Their voices rose ever higher in competition.

The bird let out a warbling song to drown them out. Her voice echoed in the jungle as she spiraled ever higher, eventually reaching high above the island once more.

"This is an amazing view!" said Jaina.

"Yes, it is." Bird tucked her wings and dove once more. "But sometimes you need to see from a bird's eye view up close!"

Down she flew into the jungle canopy, landing upon a high branch.

The wind caressed her feathers as she preened her wing, and then looked down on the world unfolding below her.

In the thick undergrowth, many creatures crawled, each with a voice of its own.

A furry anteater hummed its slow, ponderous song as it wandered lazily through the brush, long tongue flicking out of its long face. The anteater stopped and looked up at Bird as she sang down to it.

"Good…morning…" said the anteater, it is every word drawn out and rolling.

"It is a good morning!" said Bird. "But there are no ants up here, my friend."

"That's…okay." The anteater plodded along on its search.

A soft croak drew her attention, followed by another, and another.

Small frogs with very vibrant coloring hopped up the tree trunk.

112

Bird knew better than to test them: they were beautiful but dangerous if you were careless, much like the sweetest of dreams.

One of the frogs, neon green with red sides, leaped from the tree as a wind sighed through the palm fronds. The frog spread into wings of luminous glass, a butterfly with glowing blue and black patterns on its wings.

As Bird and Jaina watched the butterfly shattered into a hundred tiny slivers of blue light, and each grew wings, a sudden swarm of sky-blue butterflies shining in the shaded forest canopy.

Laughing, Bird flew down to join them, and suddenly found herself caught within a cloud of swirling blue. They spiraled with the wind, down nearly to the ground and then back up into the branches, pushing through the leaves and emerging into the sunlight beyond.

As the butterflies flew, a symphony of fluttering notes filled the air. The bird stopped flapping her wings and for a moment just drifted up on the music of the island itself: the rush of wings, wind, and waves, all joining together to create a warm sound.

The frond-leaves were as wings, emerald feathers joining her in flight. Whole flocks rose out of the green to take to the sky with her, and they soared so high even the wind envied them.

Blue skies opened up before them, and to Jaina's delight, she found they soared higher still. Into kingdoms of cloud they flew, where mountains of mist and moisture rolled past, and visions of the ancient world rose up and fell away in mere moments.

Clouds became like islands in the sky, floating upside down in an airy ocean.

The wind rolled through it all like oceanic currents, some warm and lazy, some cool and swift.

The flock changed again, leaves borne upon the wind, now clad in white cloud-feathers, wreathed in the scent of rain.

Thunder rolled and the islands gave way to a downpour, cascading from the clouds as waterfalls.

The flock dove into the rain, becoming like fish of sea green, fins like wings, but the music never changed. The song of the island: that of sea and sky, where the voices of the waves and the dreams of the wind combined.

Therefore, down they fell, back into the water, bursting through the surface and emerging from a geyser of bubbles in yet another world. There the deep blue embraced them, warm and salty, and they sank into its liquid softness. Currents enveloped them.

Colorful ocean fish darted back and forth amid the reefs that surrounded the island, and the flock changed yet again, becoming like them, bright and quick, yet trailing seaweed from their tails. Longer and longer, the trails grew, as they flew through the water around the island, binding it in green.

The land became green beneath them, and the clouds of fish were as clouds in the sky, glimpsed through the shimmering surface above them.

Green seaweed beds settled onto coral and melted together into trees with palm leaves and the rocks that once adorned the reef hung from the trees like coconuts.

Sun shone through the surface, upon which the shadows of swaying trees danced.

She landed beside a pool in the center of it all that slowly filled up with clear gleaming water.

The bird looked into the pool and Jaina was there beside her, staring at their reflections.

114

She sat back and laughed. "That was amazing!

I never knew the island was so perfectly poised between the two worlds."

"Three," said Bird cheerily.

"Earth, sea, and sky. This little island offers them all for those who want them. Even for one who has hopped and flown every single inch of this island. Do you see now why I never tire of it? To nap here would be divine, but if this whole place is like a dream come to life, would you need to?"

Jaina sat back on her hands. The warm tropical air stirred her hair and tasted faintly of salt. She smiled.

"I think it would be hard to tell the difference. This entire place is perfect. As you said, it's got something for everyone."

A coconut fell and rolled down a little sandy hill, bumping lightly into her knee.

Jaina picked it up and found that it already had a straw in it, drawn from the little reeds that surrounded the pool.

She sipped at the sweet coconut milk, the taste rolling over her tongue like the white clouds through which they had flown. Jaina lay back on a bed of soft, fragrant tropical flowers.

Closing her eyes and just relishing the tastes of the island, Jaina did not even notice the coconut slip from her fingers.

The birds continued their endless cries around her, and the wind continued to caress the waves.

Jaina fell into dreams that were little different from the waking beauty that was the island life.

CHAPTER 21

San Miguel de Allende

In the quaint town of San Miguel de Allende in the heart of Mexico, there is a neighborhood of colonial-style buildings lining narrow cobblestone roads with two thousand doors, framed by handcrafted ironwork. These doors lead to two thousand courtyards of varying sizes hidden behind the orange, yellow, and ochre facades of the street ways. The preserved cobblestone roads take the residents to a number of churches, one, in particular, is the most photographed church in Mexico, the La Parroquia de San Miguel Arcángel was built in 1880 by a native bricklayer and self-taught architect, drawing inspiration from lithographs of the grand gothic churches of Europe. The imaginative interpretation of the designs created a charming homage to the style instead of a direct replica, giving the building a unique presence. The church stretches tall, with arches and columns stacked on each other, its delicate pink patterns and spires spiraling into the sky above.

San Miguel de Allende is speckled with well-preserved historic buildings as well as being a Mecca for visual and musical artists across the country. Converted churches and convents now hose art installations, exhibits, and studios, and classrooms to learn everything from painting and sculpting to dancing, acting, and music. The courtyard of the converted convent has housed the aspirations of many students and watched the dreams of many come to fruition right in the narrow streets and lush parks of the historic city. Not only a home to the talents of Mexico, San De Allende is a host to many festivals to showcase the dedication of its people to their craft. Every year the music under the Tress festival provides an opportunity for the love of music to be shared from performer to admirer.

On this sunny summer Saturday, I wander along the cobblestone streets, past a small sample of the doors hiding secret courtyards, toward one of the music under the trees' performances. The city is bursting with talent, and the festival cannot be contained in one location. Music seekers walk the city, sampling a wide variety of genres, pausing when the music reaches the depths of the heart and moving on when the melodies sweep them to the next discovery. It is a magical union between nature, musician and audience. Along my walk, I begin to hear the sweet sound of string instruments moving in unison. I follow the notes to a small park in the heart of the historic zone. Under a tree, a string quartet is lulling a small crowd into a satisfying trance. I do not recognize the song, but my heart knows it is good. I sit on the grass and enjoy the melody of strings with the strangers beside me.

I continue my musical journey through the city, finding myself at the doors of Fabrica La Aurora, an old textile mill converted to artist studios. This building has been the hub of the art community. It thrives today with workshops and studio courtyards open to the admiring public to observe the creators at work. Jewelers, furniture makers, and painters mingle together and enjoy the creative energy in the air, along with the convenience of the small cafes and restaurants that line the patio area. Wanting to witness another art form unfold before my eyes, I decided to take a break in the patio and enjoy a traditional lunch of 'Enchilada Mineras.' Corn tortillas with onion and potatoes seasoned perfectly with the warmth of chili and cumin powders cooled by ranchero cheese was served to the miners of the region after a long day's work. I enjoy my food slowly while watching a sculpture work the clay in front of them, molding the earth into their vision right before my eyes.

Another walk down another cobblestone street brings me past three young people in a band. Strumming guitar, drumming a single bongo, and one voice softly singing pleasant words to the audience. Another street brings me to a lone guitar player. Intricately strumming out a classic Spanish guitar song, gently drumming on the base of the guitar, adding depth to the song that moves two women to dance in the street. Their eyes are closed, and bodies sway gently in the breeze along to the music. Another cobblestone road and a longing in my heart guides me to a more extensive park, with rows of chairs arranged and people flowing in to find a seat. I don't know what the performance is, but something tells me to stay. I see a chair near the front, along the edges, and the entertainers fill their seats on the stage. A full orchestra files into place on the stage, they gently pick up instruments and adjust sheet music.

At last, the conductor joins them, he bows to the audience, and the quiet lull of conversation around me comes to a close. The conductor taps his stand; at once, the orchestra raises their instruments into place, and with the sweep of the conductor's arms, dozens of musicians' spark to life in unison. The notes wash over the audience, first in a powerful wave breaking through the wall between them and us, followed by the gentle sway from one section to the next. The strings have their moment, soaring smoothly into the afternoon breeze. The horns annunciate their presence and bring the energy back up. From the back, the percussionist steadily pulses outward, creating the cocoon in which the wind instruments can punctuate the piece with their sharp melodies. I am enthralled and immediately carried away with the performance, my heart soaring and falling by the skilled movement of each musician's hands. I feel inspired and grateful for this moment in time and the afternoon spent in the presence of joyful and masterful artistry.

CHAPTER 22

Corpse

Aaahhhh! From nowhere came the most murderous shout from the midnight hour Lord Darberfield's castle. Even the maids, butlers and cooks had been the residents who dwelt at the castle and they came hurrying from the bed chambers carrying their candles into their shaking hands looking light with absolute fright, almost all them had difficulty running down their spines when they noticed the damn scream. They looked at each other in puzzlement and hurried down the staircase in such pace with fascination to the Lord Darberfield's area and saw a dreadful sight an entire shock defeated everyone at the castle since they stood nevertheless their suspended eyes concentrated on the blot blooded rug and the individual's sliced of hands that was sitting around the bloodstream, however for some odd reason there was not any indication of a weapon close to the bloodstream or the other hand.

Everyone the maids were left-handed, but one of those maid's Miss Smithers Was the very first one to pop up the question since the rest of these were frozen stiff with shock 'who is blood and sliced off is that' asked Miss Simthers timidly.

Among those butlers Mr. Woods answered, 'I do not understand miss but I'm Imagining it should be somebody out this castle because everybody is here current except for the Lord'.

'Should not we call the authorities' Shouted Miss bates she had been among those cooks In the castle.

119

'No, we can not because the authorities might imagine us we all do live in the Castle and we possibly accused of ridding the body someplace and they'll down us into the police station,' responded Mr. Woods, who'd perspiration drops slowing stripping down his head.

'Where's your human body' asked Miss Stevenson she had been another maid that seemed Directly in the mad slave Mr. Hobbs.

'What can I seem like detective Colombo, " I do not understand the killer has to have Buried the human body or pitched into a river' said Mr. Hobbs, that had been constantly sarcastic even in severe cases such as these.

Once he stated that another maids and servants obtained slightly leery Of him they believed in their heads could he's been involved in the murder or was the killer.

'What are we going to perform' said Miss Betsey from the blue was one Of the most youthful maids from the castle, so she had been the person who asked the main question.

'First thing we must do is determine who is hand and blood this belongs To see whether we could wash the stains of this carpeting because if anybody comes from the castle they're likely to find suspicious and nobody feel that we're naive' Replied Mr. Woods

He was constantly kept the mind of the castle each single time when Lord Darberfield Was off on a visit or even a meeting with the queen since he had been a trusted reliable butler.

Before they went into bed each and every Individual from the castle hunted for Some more clues the murderer left and to the human body but found no weapon no additional indications of blood no additional body components inside the castle.

The following day everybody hunted for much more evidence and finding the lost body.

120

The servants went digging into the castle grounds and gardens, a few of those Cooks hunted in the maze and the butlers moved and hunted around the forests that was 10 miles from your castle, but nobody found any indications or no evidence which may help fix the investigation therefore it had been left for a puzzle since they could not locate the body to recognize the individual or the hints to learn who the killer is. The only way that they could find out whose hand and blood this is along with also the killer is by reporting on the authorities as they've forensic testing gear there.

Miss Smithers was becoming stressed and wanted to telephone Lord Darberfield because he Was off in a camping tree having an old buddy.

'I'm getting really worried I'm calling Lord Darberfield he can understand what To do about that dreadful event after all this is his castle'

'No we should not disturb him outing after he desires a miniature holiday To go away from all of the stress besides we're capable of managing this investigation ourselves with no assistance,' said Mr. Woods, who for some odd reason had gone really squeaky about the voice.

Whilst the days gone by everybody searched for the body and much more hints To track the killer down, they were wondering why Lord Daberfield has not returned in the camping trip as he was just going for a couple of days and it's been two weeks because he has not return. So, the servants chose to ring him up despite Mr. Woods's approval. For some odd reason Lord Daberfield did not reply.

The days shortly passed months and the weeks shortly passed and Nobody has noticed Lord Daberfield and everyone had given up hunt for the body. But today they were careful in safety of this castle ensuring that no stranger or an undesirable guest penetrates the castle grounds.

They had a sinking feeling He could be dead since They went into the Mountains to the time where he'd last camped and had been no where available, the citizens hunted outside of those hills inquired passerby's nobody had seen him or even his friend Count Darcy, several servants started to believe he and his friend have disappeared with out one hint.

Possessing the castle into themselves, they had been free and did exactly what they wanted to Do this other were happy though the citizens did miss out Lord Daberfield because he had been a type lord constantly considerate to the servants and butlers and thankful he was not egotistical at all although he had been filthy rich and had no spouse but not each the inhabitants but that one.

1 afternoon Mr. Woods chose to go to the forests he attracted a scoop with him, He went deeply into the forests and began digging directly at the middle of the entire woods he dug and dug until he'd detected a leg along with a tie that seemed to belong to Lord Daberfield, therefore he had been the individual who'd been killed and his body had been buried in the core of his forests. Just how did Mr. Woods understand where the body has been, and also for what possible motive did he need to dig this up for. Now it had been Lord Daberfield's birthdaycake. He was likely to be 64 years old and Mr. Woods desired to provide a final gift to him. He climbed, and if handing him the increased he stated, 'Happy Birthday Lord Daberfield, love your ceaseless sleep and yet another thing thanks so much for your cash along with your castle'.

Mr. Woods subsequently dug up him and gave a wicked wicked laugh; he had been the Murder of Lord Daber area. Lord Daberfield was at his town that night after his butler came from the blue he made out a gun of his pocket and did not hesitate to shoothe took him three occasions and in his hands that came off, and the shout was subsequently discovered so he'd thrown the body across the window and it landed on the top of the compilation that he then proceeded upstairs and acted stunned and amazed as the remaining inhabitants were another day that he took the human body and buried it in the woods and also told a lie into the servants, maids and hamburgers he hunted for the entire body in the forests. So, you find the murder of Lord Daberfield was planned with a single wicked butler that was after a loyal butler and Lord Daberfields favored as well as a pal of his own.

And What's worse is the servants, maids and cooks did not even Have a hint it had been him and him that had murdered Lord Daberfield so no one knew that the killer actually was and they won't ever understand.

CHAPTER 23

Keeping Up Appearances

J eff shoved a bagel into his mouth as he ran out the door. If he was late again, Mr. Stevenson would have his head on a platter. He was sure there was nothing he could say or do to convince him there was a good enough reason for him to be late for three days in a row.

He hustled down the street and tried to flag down a taxi. Catching the train at this point would only serve to make him late, so he would eat the extra fare and get there with a couple of minutes to spare. He stepped into the street and held up his hand to hail the next cab that drove his way. The next one that came down the road, however, didn't stop. Perhaps they had a fare and forgot to flip the switch for the light on top of their cab.

He stood by the side of the road with his hand up, looking for the next nearest cab, which also didn't stop. With so little success on finding a cab that would take him to work and his phone telling him that he was running out of time, he decided to hit the bricks and make his way to the office on foot. If he really hustled, he might be able to get there right on time. He was familiar with the saying, "If you're right on time, then you're late," but that phrase had never quite sat well with him.

If you were right on time, then you were right on time. Being right on time couldn't mean that you were late, because you were… Well, right on time. Sure, he understood that the meaning was intended to inspire people to arrive at work with time to spare so they could prepare themselves for the day ahead and that, when the clock struck nine, they were ready to do their best to do a job well-done while on company time. However, the company didn't pay him to be early. They paid him

124

from nine in the morning to five in the evening, and those were the hours between which he would be available for work and prepping for work activities.

Just as Jeff began to find himself really deep in thought, he realized that he had arrived at the office. He jogged through the door and up the stairs and arrived at his desk promptly at nine in the morning. He heaved a sigh of relief, put his bag and his jacket on the hook in his office and sat down to begin working.

"Hey, Jeff I need you to—" Jeff looked up at Mr. Stevenson, who stood in the doorway to his office looking at him disappointedly.

"What, what's wrong?" Jeff asked, alarmed.

"Katie, can you come here a second?" Mr. Stevenson asked someone outside Jeff's office. When the spritely girl walked up to him, Mr. Stevenson said something to her quietly. She took her phone out of her pocket and focused on it for a moment.

Seconds later, Jeff's phone began to ring in his pocket. He took it out and saw that it was Katie calling him. Perplexed, he stared at it for a moment before calling out to them.

"Is this some kind of joke? What's going on here?" They didn't answer him, so he picked up his phone. "… Hello?" He saw Mr. Stevenson take the phone from her and take a few steps away.

"Jeff, this is the third day in a row that you haven't been on time for work. If I don't see a significant improvement in your performance, I'm going to have to—"

"Mr. Stevenson, I'm right behind you, in my office. You looked right at me before asking Katie to call me for you. Did you honestly not see me? You looked right at me." There was a long pause.

"What are you talking about?" Mr. Stevenson turned back around and walked back to Jeff's office door. "I'm looking in your office right now and it's empty.

"Well, I have no idea how that's possible, as I'm looking at you right now while you're talking to me. You're wearing a blue shirt today and a purple tie. Looks new." Jeff waved at him exaggeratedly, but he could tell from the movements of Mr. Stevenson's eyes that he wasn't registering that Jeff was in front of him at all.

"Are you playing a prank on me right now?" Mr. Stevenson asked quietly. "If you are, I really don't think this is funny."

"Scouts honor, I am being completely truthful with you. You're not playing some kind of joke on me, are you? I'm sitting here waving at you and you're honestly telling me that you cannot see me?"

"I am honestly telling you that all I see in your office is furniture." Jeff paused for a moment.

"Look on the hook behind the door. Can you see my bag and jacket?" Mr. Stevenson walked into the office and closed the door. He put the phone back up to his ear.

"Yes, I see them. Did you leave those here last night?"

"No, I put them there three minutes ago when I came in for work. I sat down at my desk and seconds later, you walked in to ask me to do something. That's when you called Katie to come over, then she called me, and now here we are. You can't hear me talking either? I'm in the room with you right now and talking at pretty full volume, yet you can't hear me?"

"I can only hear you through the phone." Jeff could tell that Mr. Stevenson was reluctantly answering his questions and that he was still mostly sure that he was being played for a fool.

126

"Okay, so it seems like the things that I am touching are the only things that are missing. Can you see a bagel anywhere in the office?" Mr. Stevenson looked around.

"No, I don't see any bagels." Jeff set his bagel on the desk.

"How about now?" Mr. Stevenson's eyes immediately snapped to the desk as soon as Jeff set down the bagel. They widened and the color drained out of his face as he whispered, What in God's name…

"I don't know, but I sure would like to. Mr. Stevenson, I don't know what the hell is going on here and I'm starting to get scared."

"Call me Hal. I want to try something. This is nuts."

"Okay, Hal… What did you have in mind?" Hal picked up a stress ball that Jeff kept on a nearby shelf.

"I want to see what happens when you catch this. Where are you?"

"I'm sitting in the chair." Hal lobbed the stress ball to Jeff, who caught it easily. Hal's eyes widened again when the ball seemed to slip through midair and into nothingness. Jeff looked at the ball that sat plainly in his hands. "Did that go the way you expected it to?"

"I would say 'expected' is a strong word, but I had a hunch. As soon as you caught the ball, it completely disappeared. Anything you're wearing or holding is completely obscured from view. Put the ball back on the desk." Jeff did as he was told, and he watched Hal's eyes light up as the ball slipped back into view.

"I have no idea what to do with this information. Are you the only one who can't see me?" Hal looked at the chair in wonder.

"That's a great question. Okay, wait here. I'm giving Katie her phone back and I'll call you on mine." Hal all but ran out of the office to find his phone in his office. He came back with his headset in his ears. Clearly, Hal was ready to test the limits of this anomaly.

127

Hal called Jeff's phone and directed him to walk out of his office and into the lane that ran down the center of the cubicles in the main work floor. He told Jeff to walk to the entrance of the first cubicle and ask the person inside it if they were having a good morning.

"Hello, Janet. Are you having a good morning?" There was a long pause, during which Janet sat at her computer, typing a letter to a vendor. "Janet, are you having a good morning?" Nothing from Janet. "Janet, no one likes your quiche." Still no response from Janet.

"Good one. This is going to take all morning if you go from cube to cube, asking everyone things and insulting them."

"All right, it was a joke, Hal. What do you suggest instead?"

"Stand in the middle of the lane and yell that there's free cake in the conference room. Anyone who hears that is bound to leap up immediately."

"It's 9:15 in the morning. I'll say donuts."

"Ah yes, acceptable breakfast cake."

"Save it for your blog." Jeff stood at the center of the lane and shouted. "THERE ARE FREE DONUTS IN THE CONFERENCE ROOM. ANYONE WHO CAN HEAR THIS ANNOUNCEMENT SHOULD MEET ME IN THERE, RIGHT NOW."

Jeff craned his neck and looked around at the cubicles that surrounded him. No one moved a muscle or said anything. He turned to look at Hal, who stared in the general area of where Jeff stood.

"Well, I think it's safe to say that no one can see or hear you." Jeff paused for a moment.

"Yeah, I guess they can't. What the hell do I do now?"

"I think this, counts as a good enough reason for you to take the rest of the day off. Maybe see… A physicist? I have no idea."

128

"Thanks, I'll try that." Jeff grabbed his jacket, bag, and bagel and left the office. He took care not to bump into anyone on the way home, as he had no idea what would happen.

He got home and sat on his sofa, trying to think of who to contact or what to do. Before he could come up with any answers, however, he dozed off in the comfortable warmth of his couch cushions.

He awoke about an hour later to his phone ringing. Spam call from an auto-dialer. He ignored it and sat up straight. He decided he would take his phone to the park and research this kind of anomaly to see if anyone had any information to offer.

Just as he was exiting his building, someone on a bicycle was headed toward him.

"Comin' through," the boy riding it called as he swerved to avoid hitting Jeff.

"Stupid kid," Jeff said. "Wait." He whipped his head to look after the boy, but he was long gone.

A man was passing by on the sidewalk and Jeff called to him. "Excuse me, sir." The man stopped and looked at Jeff. Jeff paused, considering how odd it would seem for him to ask if he could see him. "Have you got the time?"

"Oh, yes it's half-past eleven."

"Thank you, sir." Jeff nodded and walked the other way to end his interaction with the man. Was it really so simple as that? A nap reset the anomaly completely.

Jeff wondered if it would ever happen again, or if he would need to spend the first hour or so of every day, trying to find out if others could see him or not.

CHAPTER 24

Down the Prehistoric Rabbit Hole

Alternative introduction:

A s I read this and begin to drift comfortably asleep, I don't know whether I will find myself drifting asleep more to the sound of my voice or the words I read, or perhaps to the spaces between the words. And as I drift comfortably asleep I'll just read this story to myself."

As you comfortably begin to drift off to sleep, I don't know whether you will drift deeper with the sound of my voice, or whether it will be with the spaces between my words, or whether it will be that you drift deeper and more comfortably asleep with the words that I use. And so, as you drift comfortably asleep, I'm just going to tell you a story in the background. And while I tell that story you can fall asleep comfortably.

There was a girl out in her garden one day. She was playing and running around and then she had the most unusual experience, while she was playing she saw a rabbit hole. It was an unusually large rabbit hole, so she went over to that hole and peered inside. It was dark, so she decided to crawl inside a little bit to get a better look. As she crawled in she noticed the hole got larger and larger, until eventually the hole was large enough for her to stand up and walk in. And as she walked along the inside of this rabbit hole, so she noticed that it turned from having mud all around the sides, to merging into having concrete or some other manmade materials all around the sides, which gradually merged into looking like a corridor, with flat sides, a flat roof, an echoey concrete floor and a glow at the end of this corridor which continued to get brighter as she walked closer to it with curiosity. She reached out with

130

her hand and ran her fingers over the wall, curious about the way the wall seemed to turn from mud into concrete. She was aware of the way her footsteps were now echoing down the corridor and she could look back and see that rabbit hole and yet when she looked forward, it looked like there was a glow at a door, or something off in the distance.

And with a sense of calm curiosity she walked her way towards that door and when she arrived at that door she saw that it looked like a lift, she pressed the button next to the door and waited and waited and she could hear movement behind the door, the sound of a lift descending and she waited and waited and then with a ping, the door slid open and she walked inside the lift. And she thought that this was a very peculiar situation, a very strange thing to happen, she saw that there were five levels and decided that she would just go all the way to the bottom and so she pressed one.

She waited a moment as the door slid shut and the lift began to lower, from five, to four, to three and she could see light passing by the lift as the movement continued to happen, to two, to one, where the lift stopped and the door slid open. She walked out of the lift and found herself in a vast cavern, as if somehow this lift had taken her down into a cave. She wondered whether this cave was underneath her back garden, because she didn't know anything about this. She started exploring. Walking around the outside of the cave initially, touching the cave wall, getting a feel for it, hearing the occasional drip of water echoing through the cave, hearing the way her footsteps echoed around the cave. She couldn't hear any other noises in the cave. After a while, she saw something that looked a bit different in the cave wall. Something that looked like it was artificial but made to blend in, made to look like part of the cave.

She pushed against this artificial area and pulled on it and felt around it, trying to find any clue. Eventually she knocked into a stone on the floor and realized that although it looked like it was a stone that should have moved, just like a loose stone or pebble, it didn't go anywhere, so she kicked it again and noticed it still didn't go anywhere. She lent down,

felt around on that stone and realized that it was like a lever that could
be pulled upwards. She pulled that stone upwards, let go and it popped
back down into place. And as it did, the wall beside her slid backwards
and disappeared, opening up a secret tunnel. And she walked into this
secret tunnel, feeling curiouser and curiouser the deeper she went into
the experience and the weirdest thing happened, as she was approaching
the end of the tunnel, so everything started to get lighter as if she was
walking towards daylight. And she continued walking and she started
hearing the sounds of birds and the sounds of other animals she didn't
recognize. And she could feel a breeze on her face and she exited the
tunnel and realized she was partway up a cliff overlooking a vast valley
with trees and grasses and above looked like a sky with clouds and yet
she was aware that she was inside the ground and this must be a huge
cave and she couldn't understand how the ceiling here is glowing like
normal daylight. She couldn't see where the sun was, but it looked as
normal as when she is outside in the woods normally.

She saw that there was a path down to the bottom of the valley and she
followed that path and she could feel the breeze on her face. She could
smell the woodland smell, smell the wood and plants, hear the animals.
Then as she looked around in the valley, she noticed something she
didn't initially believe and had to double check. It looked like there were
dinosaurs in this valley. There were pterodactyls in the sky, and it was
like a prehistoric world and some of the plants had vast flat leaves,
others looked like unusual conifers. And apart from grasses, there didn't
seem to be very many flowers that she could see. She was fascinated by
this; somehow, she had found her way to a prehistoric world and she
started exploring in this prehistoric world, climbing up a tree, watching
as giant dinosaurs walked past. Really getting absorbed in this
prehistoric world.

Then she noticed, off in the distance, by a lake, it looked like there was
a person there. So, she decided she wanted to go and talk with them and
find out what this place is. She climbed down from the tree and carefully
worked her way through the valley, she had this feeling like everything

132

was perfectly fine and safe, but she wanted to be careful, nonetheless. So, she walked down the valley, breathing in the smells, feeling the grass and the air on her face, noticing the sound of each footstep. And as she continued down the valley, she could see the person was just milling around, doing something at the lake and she got closer and closer and noticed that they looked like they were a scientist and eventually she managed to get to where they were. And she kept just out of sight and watched them working and they were testing the water and taking a sample and they were testing the air and writing down some notes. They were taking a few pictures and they were wheeling something, and they put their samples on the thing they were wheeling, and they started heading around the outside of the lake. The girl carefully and quietly followed and watched as they reached the cabin and went into the cabin and she wondered whether she should follow, whether she should knock on the cabin door and introduce herself.

After a little while she decided that is what she would do, she had to know what this place was, she had her curiosity and she wanted to know and so she knocked on the door and she could see through the window that the person appeared startled, but they came to the door and they saw the girl stood there. They asked who she was, how she had found them and why she was here? She said "Those were the questions I was going to ask you. Who are you? Why are you here? Where is here?"

The person invited her in. She sat down in that cabin and could feel a certain coolness and comfort inside the cabin. She asked him, "Where is here and who are you?"

And they wanted to know the same from her. They explained that they created this place, they have spent their life creating this place. They have had a fascination with the prehistoric world, with saving things and they had managed years earlier to create this prehistoric world underground and they are the master of this world. Their role is to watch over it, to do as little as possible without interfering with it, but just monitor it and make sure it ticks along okay.

133

And the girl found this interesting. She said that she had got there by following a rabbit hole and the master realized that somehow, maybe a rabbit, maybe a different animal had obviously burrowed into the ground and had somehow managed to burrow into one of the corridors of this base, this underground facility. So, this curious girl had followed that into this underground facility, and she had so many questions about it, about how it was made, about the size of it, about how they have recreated the sun. How they make sure there is enough oxygen and the correct composition of the air and that the plants can grow and where they got all of these prehistoric plants and animals. The scientist explained everything, they normally didn't talk to anyone, so they enjoyed having someone who was interested in all of this who they could talk to about it all. They talked about how this was a secret place that no-one was to know about. The girl swore that she would also keep it secret. They said, this is somewhere they find a sense of wonder and serenity, a sense of peace, a sense of being back to a time before lots of chaos. To a simpler time. They explained about how they enjoy relaxing by the lake, just doing their job, gathering some samples, feeding that information back, relaxing in the cabin. Watching dinosaurs, pterodactyls and other animals going about their lives. Just as they would have done millions and millions of years earlier.

They find that this is their safe place, this is their place away from the hustle and bustle of the 'real world' and when they go home they have to hear cars and traffic and have lots of chaos and yet here they can enjoy peace and serenity and have a sense of wonder. The girl appreciated all of this. But, she also realized that she was away from home and as far as anyone thought, she was playing in the garden, but now she has played far out of the garden. So, she left the cabin, she was told that if she kept it a secret she could come and visit again. She left the cabin, wandered back through the valley, climbed up to that secret tunnel, she followed that secret tunnel and found her way back to the lift. And then back to the corridor and then eventually back to her garden. She sat down in her garden, relaxing under a tree, thinking about the experience she had just had and while she relaxed there thinking about the experience she had just had, her mind drifted and dreamed and floated off as she comfortably and relaxed, fell asleep.

CHAPTER 25

The Place of Greatest Comfort

W elcome your breath as you find your relaxed state of mind and body.

Let your energy flow freely into your choice to let go, lie down, take comfort, and find solitude in the night hours, or before a long rest.

Prepare your body, your thoughts, your emotions, to fall forward into relief and inner comfort.

Let your soul feel prepared to feel held warmly by loving energy and inner light.

Take a few deep breaths in and exhales out to align with your comfort.

Help your body feel snuggled in and at peace.

Find all of the soft cushions and blankets you need to feel at home and at peace.

You are going to become more and more relaxed with every breath you take.

With every inhale, refresh your body with new oxygen, new energy, cleansing, and purifying your inner world.

With every exhale, release all of the tension from your body and your thoughts.

Release your worries and concerns.

Breathe in comfort, peace of mind, serenity.

KATHERINE BENNETT

Breathe out stress and worry, negativity, and pain.

As you connect further to your relaxed state of mind, feel soothed and nurtured by your choice to take time for a bedtime story.

Acknowledge that you are taking good care of yourself right now, at this moment.

Acknowledge that you are nurturing yourself back to health and giving yourself space to heal and rejuvenate.

Going deeper into this restful state, connect to your warmest memories of home, your most filling spaces you've known.

Connect to your places of greatest comfort in your mind and start to see in your third eye what that space looks like.

Open your heart and your mind to the part of your wholeness that feels the safest, the most comfortable, the most nurtured.

It could be your childhood home, or perhaps the space you live in now.

Maybe it is a beloved holiday memory or a film that gives you comfort.

It may be as simple as a picture in your mind of an old country cottage with a crackling fire and a pot of stew simmering on the stove.

Let your mind form this place of greatest comfort.

Take a few moments, breathing in slowly, letting it out steadily, and picture this serene and wholesome place...

You are here to find solace and inner harmony.

This dwelling space you are in that feels comforting to you is where you have come to feel at ease.

This is where you can become well again, nurtured, warmed by the fire.

This is where you will be fed by loved ones, family friends, or even your spiritual guides who have come to hold space for you.

137

When you take a look around this space, who is here to give you comfort?

What energies have come to support you and keep you safe and warm?

It can be anyone.

It can be anything.

Let your subconscious mind welcome whatever comes to give you balance and inner peace...

Continue to lay in this space, snuggled into your warm blankets, cozy and comforted as you welcome these energies, whether they are people or spirits.

What does it feel like to be surrounded by a warm, loving company?

How does it feel to have a place just to lay down and be taken care of?

You have no obligations here, no one to take care of.

You are the one being cared for.

You are the one who is being nurtured and loved.

Let the spirits and people who have traveled to this place in your heart gather around you and give you love and attention.

Feel their soft, friendly smiles giving you comfort and openness in your soul and mind.

As you continue to rest in the space of great comfort, the people, friends, allies, spirit guides, or others who have come to nurture and care for you are beginning to prepare a feast of the most nutritious and nourishing food.

All of your favorite foods that will heal you and make you feel whole are there.

You can hear the sound of foods being chopped, the sound of boiling soup on the stove, the aroma of fresh ingredients.

They are here to help you feel well and loved.

They are roasting things in the oven, the smell filling the whole space.

They are stirring the logs on the fire and making sure your blankets are tucked in.

Keeping you warm and cozy.

You have everything you need here.

You can just be.

You are being taken care of and loved in this place of greatest comfort.

The feeling that surrounds you is that of being held by all of the things that make you feel warm, whole, heart-felt, and secure.

The foods that are being prepared are the ones that make you feel nurtured and nourished.

The pleasantness of this place is what feels so healing and good.

It is your inner home and that good feeling that comes from your wholeness within.

As you are laying there, swaddled in blankets, taking in the aroma of your favorite dishes being prepared and the sounds of laughter and loving energy coming from those who have gathered, you feel someone lift you up and carry you, wrapped in warmth, to a table where there are many places laid for you and all of your company to share a delicious meal by a warm, glowing fire.

As you look from one end of the table to the other, it feels endless.

The candles are lit.

There is food on every inch of the table: fresh-baked bread, still hot from the oven, bowls of fresh fruits and herbs, homemade cookies, goblets of delicious drinks, roasted dishes, everything your heart desires, laid out in front of you.

You are surrounded by the love and affection of whoever is here with you.

The fire is crackling, and someone adds another log to keep it going.

As you look around the table at the feast, at your family and friends, your spiritual guides, you are filled with a sense of warmth and wonder.

There is nothing but kindness and generosity here, and you have no other concerns.

Everyone is merry and filling up on the wonderfully nutritious and nourishing foods.

You feel at peace, connected to this moment, to these friends and allies, to this meal.

When you have finished eating, and you glance around the table, you can sense and feel the contentedness of those around you, and it fills your heart with joy and tenderness.

You are warm in your blankets, full of the glorious feast, and held by the family that surrounds you.

You are free just to relax and breathe for a few moments, taking in this feeling of true peace and serenity.

Just as you feel like you could drift off to sleep, you feel someone lift you up again and carry you over to a soft, cushioned sofa near the fire.

You are tucked gently into your blankets, swaddled like a baby as the others gather around the sitting place near the fire.

Everyone is together for a delightful story to help everyone drift off into a safe and comfortable world of dreams.

140

You listen to the story as it begins.

Nothing feels more pleasant than having this comfort, this warmth, this generosity of spirit.

You can sense the blissfulness of everyone gathering together for a story to continue relaxing and feeling connected to the place of greatest comfort.

Your breath is slow and steady and deep.

You have nothing to think about or control in this place.

You have nothing to worry about, no problems to solve.

You are free just to relax and exist in the warmth of this space with these loving energies holding and embracing you.

As the story begins to unfold, you feel a release from deep within that lets you know that you are free to fall asleep anytime you feel like it.

You are welcome to listen until your body and mind float away, deeper and deeper into the world of dreams, into total relaxation and healing.

The story begins to take shape in your ears as you snuggle tightly into your covers, surrounded by the warm, healing light of the fire and the sense that you are not alone, that you are protected by those that surround you.

It begins as you take a deep breath in and sigh it out with relief...

Once upon a time, there was a cottage nestled deep in a forest.

The forest was very old, and the trees had been listening to all of the life within the forest for thousands of years.

The cottage had been there for a long time too, and tonight it was full of love and warmth and serenity.

The people inside of the cottage were baking loaves of bread and sweets, stirring a large pot of stew, and feasting on the delicious flavors of the

Autumn time as the nights grew colder and the wind blew harder, whispering of the winter to come.

The feast was fragrant and sumptuous.

The taste of every bite was fulfilling.

Every nibble of soft, warm bread felt soothing to the soul; every sip of hot broth was warming to the heart.

The candles burned and the warm glow of firelight permeated to simple cottage walls, giving peace and comfort to all who sat at the table.

All around, there was laughter and kindness and friendship.

All around, there was life and beauty, and harmony.

The people sitting at the table felt satiated and at peace.

It was that time when all the food has been eaten and all the bellies are full when the gathering of life finds the comfort of a story to close the night.

When the feast was finished, the people gathered around the fire, along with all of the animals that were there to be peaceful and warm and gentle in front of the fire.

Someone began to tell a story, as everyone covered themselves in warm blankets, full of food at the feast's end...

The storyteller gathered their voice and came to a spot by the fire, and in soft, gentle, soothing tones began to tell a story that would send everyone off into a dream, and the story went something like this...

Once upon a time, there was a place of greatest comfort.

And no matter where you are in this world, you can find it.

All you have to do is close your eyes, take a nice deep breath, and remember this place that you know in your heart.

It is the place where the feat is always being made, where the fire is always warm, where the friends are always close by to wrap you in their arms and soothe you into a loving slumber.

This place is ancient and old, and yet it is fresh and new.

You have seen it in your dreams and in your daytime, too.

It is everywhere and nowhere; it is always by your side.

It is within your very nature, this story of heart and mind.

This place of greatest comfort is the story you will tell, every night when you go to sleep and find the place that suits you well.

This story is ongoing and will take you very far, deep into your dreamworld, to the farthest star.

Just gaze into the fire and hear the words unfold.

This is the place of greatest comfort, the greatest story ever told.

The whole world knows this story for we all have it in our hearts, to find our inner peace in a cottage safe at night.

All around the forest, deep to river's edge, down below the valley, in every cave, behind every rock, along the highest ledge, all the creatures are resting and feeling comfort under the night sky.

There is a community in the nighttime, and family of night.

There are always those around you, falling deeper into sleep- every animal, every bird, all of the people around you by the fire who hear the story in the place of greatest comfort.

The story drifts away from you as you ink deeper into relaxation and calm.

You have never felt so comfortable, so take care of, so whole.

The words from the story are faint and distant now.

143

You can hear it through your quiet mind as you breathe in deeply and feel the sublime joy of rest and comfort tonight.

You sink even more deeply into the blankets and the cushions as the storyteller's voice becomes a part of your dream.

You are fully relaxed now and can let go of everything.

There is only this place for you now, this place of greatest comfort.

You are taken care of, loved, and held.

You are able to heal from this space, as you sleep, as you dream.

Your place of greatest comfort is always here for you and will always keep you safe and warm and protected as you trust your mind and body to fully release and relax, deep into your slumber.

Goodnight…sweet dreams…may your story continue tomorrow.

CHAPTER 26

Water for the Queen

There once was a young knight named Pip, and Pip admired his queen. The Queen of Alanstar was one of the fairest women in the land. She had a mature demeanor, but creamy white skin, and long-flowing, silky black hair that seemed to envelop her throne. After the King passed many moons ago, the Queen ruled the land with a fair amount of care.

One day, the Queen summoned Pip to her throne room. The young knight bowed to his queen.

"What do you desire?" he asked.

"Good afternoon, my dear knight. I'm currently low on drinking water, and the knights who normally bring it to me are taking the day off."

Pip scratched his head a bit. There was plenty of water around. But before he could ask, the Queen answered for him.

"I drink the water from the peak of the Wellspring Mountain. At its tip, the cleanest, clearest water known to man resides. They say a fairy lives on top of the mountain, purifying the water. As it goes down the mountain, it becomes a little less pure, but still drinkable. However, I desire only the cleanest water the land has to offer. Could you give me a pail of it?"

Pip nodded. All his work for the Queen so far had been to mop up the castle, or to change her bed covers. This was something that maybe, just maybe, she'd reward him with.

145

The Queen handed him an empty pail, complete with a lid. This golden pail had some jewels in its rims, and it looked a little tacky, but shimmered, nonetheless. Pip immediately set forth after some preparations. He put everything on his trusted steed, Pap. Pap was a beautiful white horse who served him well in the few years he had been a night. With Pap by his side, Pip told him to giddy-up, and they were off, away from the castle's stables and to the unknown.

The Wellspring Mountain was not too far from the Kingdom of Alanstar. Its water, minerals, and wildlife all nourished the kingdom quite well. With that said, there was still a bit of travel before he made it to the kingdom, so Pip trotted down the field, seeing all the sights.

A few farmers began the harvest, picking up pumpkins, corn, and all those other delicious foods. It was almost relaxing watching them. However, Pip knew that time was of the essence, and he continued forward.

However, his stomach growled. He reached into his satchel, and to his gasps, no food was in it. He then realized there was a hole in the satchel, and all his trail mix he brought came out like breadcrumbs. He sighed and stopped at one of the farms. There, he saw a young woman harvesting some corn. She was a freckled-face woman with hair the color and shape of the corncobs she was picking.

"Hello," Pip said. "I am Pip." He explained his situation as briefly as he could, knowing that a country girl probably didn't have much interest in the doings of the kingdom. However, she did listen with a keen ear.

"I'm Pop," the woman said, a smile flashing. "I was just harvesting a bit for my father before he got home. If you want a piece of corn, you can have it."

She smiled at Pip and handed him a piece of corn. He bit into it. Crunchy and sweet, it tasted just as good as cooked corn that had been lightly salted and buttered.

146

"Thank you for that," Pip said, and with that, he took off, but not before leaving a few coins as a reward. Pop tried to call out for him, but he just continued on his journey. She seemed like a nice woman, but he had one queen in his sights.

After an hour's worth of travel, he saw the Wellspring Mountain, with it looking like a painted picture in the distance. Water traveled through its peak, and Pip watched the stream as it went all the way down. At the very least, the stream would be easy to travel, but it was still quite annoying to think about.

Pap ran towards the mountain, and as they arrived at the foot, the horse let out a sad whinny. The mountain was steep, but Pap looked at his owner, knowing he had to make the climb.

And so, their journey up the Wellspring Mountain began. The sound of the stream brought some relief, calming Pip's racing mind. Despite the climb, this task seemed safe. The scariest threat Pip faced so far was black bear that lapped up some water out of the mountain, but that bear just looked at Pip and paid no mind. The water seemed to have a calming effect towards nature, and Pip and Pap stopped a few times to taste the mountain's water. It was already so clear, clean, and tasty. The Queen must have been really picky about her water.

Despite the initial climb being a bit of a breeze, the mountain soon began to steepen. There was a point where Pap made a sad whinney, unable to go any further. Pip hopped off.

"You just stay here," he said to Pap. "And I'll handle the rest."

He tied Pap next to a stream, leaving some oats behind. Pip unloaded any unneeded gear he had expect for his mountain climb, keeping only the pail, his equipment needed to climb, and the corn that Pop gave him. It was a long piece of corn, and quite filling. He munched on a bit as he began his climb up.

147

Pip's heart beat a bit as he climbed up, going higher and higher, his axe sinking into the mountainside. The cool, fall day soon became one that was a bit chillier the higher he went. The cool breeze danced around his temple and made his teeth chatter a bit, but he continued to climb.

As he climbed, with only his thoughts to entertain him, his mind began wandering. He was a kid again, training with his friends, their swords connecting in a rhythm that made him smile as he thought about it some more.

At the time, both him and his friend, Jaq, who since had departed for the Kingdom of Pio, always declared their love for the queen. "I'll be the queen's bodyguard!" Pip declared.

"No, I will," Jaq countered, and they continued to fight.

Pip chuckled as he climbed onward. He guessed this fight was still going on, even if Jaq had long since left the kingdom.

As he continued his climb, his limbs began growing weary. The soothing water coming from down the mountain could only comfort him so much. Eventually, Pip saw a cave mouth, and he climbed inside. The cave wasn't too deep, but it gave him some time to relax. Pip nibbled on the corn a bit and looked outside. It was a beautiful view from how high he was. He could see the kingdom from where he stood, along with the tower where the queen was likely enjoying herself. He smiled and took a nap. The sun changed its position and soon shined inside the mountain. He yawned, feeling a bit refreshed. Last night, he couldn't fall asleep a bit, with visions of the Queen dancing in his head. A nap was definitely what the doctor ordered.

Pip continued his ascent, the temperature growing a bit colder and colder but he still persevered. He could see his skin reddening, and a bit of snot ran down his nose, but he still climbed. The queen would love him for this; he just knew it!

148

After what seemed like an eternity, he could see the top. Pip climbed straight to the top, and there, at the apex of the mountain, he saw something that made his eyes widen.

It was a beautiful hot spring. Steam rose from it, the heat immediately ridding himself of any potential frostbite he may have had. So, these were the legendary hot springs where the kingdom got his water. Here, the water was at its purest. It was hot, but free from any dirt, toxins, and packed filled with minerals needed to keep the body going.

Pip filled up his own canteen with some of the spring water, as he'd try it himself. Then, he began filling up the pail with the water. Soon, the pail was filled up, and he screwed the lid on. The water was safe and secure, and the way down was always better than the way up. Pip was about to make his way down, when he realized something.

This was probably going to be a once in a lifetime opportunity. Why couldn't he relax a bit? Pip took off his clothes and hopped into the hot springs. The water was that perfect balance of hot, but not too scalding. He felt the minerals kiss his skin, and the steam cleanse him of anything dirty he had on it. He let himself drift off a bit, almost falling asleep at the mercy of the springs. Ah.

"Hey!"

Pip opened his eyes. In front of him, a woman the size of a ruler floated above him, translucent wings flapping. She had crystal blue eyes, hair the color of a mountain snow, and a frown on her face.

"I spent all the time purifying the water, and yet, here is a man who dares to dirty himself in the springs. You should be ashamed of yourself."

Pip rubbed his eyes. Maybe he was just seeing things, but in front of him was a

"Fairy!" he exclaimed. He stood up and hopped out, and the fairy fluttered to where he was.

149

"Of course," the fairy said. "I am the Great Pixie, and I clean up all the water. But the water won't be too clean if you contaminate it. It's going to take me hours to purify it again! You should be ashamed of yourself. I ought to turn you into a mountain toad!"

Pip gasped. "I'm sorry," was all he could mutter. "I've traveled for so long, just to fetch a pail for my queen, and I wanted to take a break."

The Great Pixie nodded. "I don't blame you, but don't do it again. Gee, though. Fetching a pail for your queen? That sounds like a whole lot of work. Is she paying you well?"

Come to think of it, Pip shook his head. "She gives me payments for cleaning her room and for doing tasks, but it's just enough to eat and nothing more."

"Then why do you do it?" the pixie asked.

Pip scratched his chin. "I do it because I love my queen."

"Yeesh," the Pixie uttered, fluttering around Pip as she shook her head. "You do realize that she isn't going to 'return the favor,' if you get what I mean, just because you did something nice for her."

"Buzz off," Pip said. "I know what I'm doing."

The Pixie shook her head again. "Men, I swear. I'm glad I'm a pixie and not one of you humans. Anyway, I suppose you should be going. Go serve your queen or whatever."

Pip opened his eyes. He was back taking a dip in the hot springs. As he stood up, he looked for all signs of the pixie. However, she was gone.

"Did I fall asleep?" he muttered. It seemed so real. The fluttering of the wings, the sassy attitude, it all seemed to happen not too long ago in a plane that resembled reality. And yet, here he was, just a fool who almost drowned in the hot springs.

With that, he put his clothes back on, grabbed his pail and canteen, and began the journey down. As expected, it was a cakewalk. He sipped from the canteen when he was about halfway down. It tasted crystal clear and as he drank it, it felt like the water was washing everything unclean from his body until what was left was a crystal-clear interior.

Pip soon reached the bottom, and there, he met Pap again and began his journey back to the kingdom. The sun began to set as he made his way to the castle. Soon, he was back at the throne room.

"I see you are back," the Queen said. "I thought you may have fallen off." She chuckled a bit as he laid the pail at her feet. She opened the pail and sipped from it.

"Crystal clear spring water," she said. "My humblest regards for you doing this for me. None of the other soldiers wanted to do it, to be honest."

Pip smiled. "So, my lady, what do I get for doing all that work for you?"

The queen tapped her foot. "Well, our budget is a bit low, but I'll try to compensate you soon. Otherwise, your work here is done."

Pip sighed. "Is there anything else you could give me?"

An awkward air filled the room. Finally, the queen opened her mouth, and the words did not calm Pip.

"Not that I know of. Anyway, I'll be returned to my quarters. See you in the morrow."

With that, she retreated, and Pip was left in an empty throne room. He accomplished the task, and the queen seemed satisfied, and yet Pip had a hole as empty as that pail would soon be when the queen was thirsty.

The pixie's words echoed in his ear. Perhaps the queen wasn't meant for him. He was much younger, and had much less power, and the queen just saw him as her errand boy.

These thoughts danced around his head as he went to bed. He closed his eyes, and despite having a bit of trouble falling asleep, the fatigue of the day soon caught up to him. He fell into a dark, dreamless, descent into sleep.

When he woke up, his stomach growled, already hungry for breakfast. He reached into his satchel and saw that he had a bit of corn to him. He munched on it, and as he did so, a knight entered his quarters. "Pip, your Highness needs you," he said.

Pip finished the corn, and then looked at the cob. With a sigh, he got dressed, but rather than go to the queen's quarters, he instead walked to the stables. Pap looked at him, yawned, and accepted his ride with ease. Pip galloped out of the kingdom and into the countryside, where he swore a fairy was chasing him. But as he looked back, there was nothing. Fairies were not real, at least, he didn't think so.

Pip traveled for what seemed like forever, and then he eventually stopped at the cornfield that lied in front of him. There, he saw Pop, tending to the corn. She picked a few ears as Pip went closer to her.

He approached Pop, and she turned around and smiled. Pip smiled back.

CHAPTER 27

The Wisdom Search

A s I read this and begin to drift comfortably asleep, I don't know whether I will find myself drifting asleep more to the sound of my voice or the words I read, or perhaps to the spaces between the words. And as I drift comfortably asleep I'll just read this story to myself."

So, as you listen to me and you comfortably begin to fall asleep, I don't know whether you will find yourself drifting comfortably to sleep to the sounds of my words, to the spaces between my words, or just listening along to my voice in the background as you fall asleep. And while you fall asleep I am just going to tell you a story about a man who enjoyed going out to sea.

Every year he would go on a trip on a boat. His favorite thing was to swim with humpback whales. Every year he would go out on a boat, he would go out to sea on that boat and he would sit on that boat in diving gear and wait. And he would wait patiently and quietly, listening to the water lapping on the side of the boat, feeling the gentle rocking of the boat as he just gazes out over the water, feeling the sea breeze on his skin, noticing what the sky looks like, gazing out towards the horizon, scanning around the horizon, scanning the water for signs of the humpback whales arriving. And every year those humpback whales seem to arrive in this location.

And so, he just sits calmly and patiently and waits and not only does he like diving with the humpback whales, but he finds the entire experience calming and relaxing, just having patience, nothing to think about or worry about. Just waiting and relaxing. And then after some time, as the sun passes across the sky, he sees a little cloud appear from the ocean. And then the dark back of a humpback whale slides just above the surface of the water and back under again, so he drives the boat closer to the whales. And the closer he gets, the more he sees of what is there. He notices that there is an adult humpback whale and a juvenile humpback whale, and he sees how calmly they are just swimming through the water. He drops the anchor and he drop into the water. He can feel that water flow into his wetsuit as he dives down under the water in his scuba gear. And he can see the size of those whales, see their slow graceful movements, hearing the whale calls. Just watching as those whales gracefully swim passed and watching how those whale's eyes appear to be so inquisitive, with such curiosity. And how the juvenile whale seems to want to come over to him and explore him. And the adult whale just keeps that juvenile at a bit of distance while assessing the diver and only after some assessing does the adult allow the juvenile and themselves to move closer.

They swim close enough for the diver to reach out with their hand and while their hand is outstretched, the juvenile swims in and rubs itself against his hand. And like all his past experiences, he feels this experience is an incredible experience, a moving experience, showing such intelligence in these whales, such love from the whales. He turns himself around weightlessly in the water, to keep tracking those whales as they swim comfortably around him. He enjoys this time in the water. Being in the water weightless with these whales, time seems to stand still. And after a while the whales take a deep breath and dive and he watches as they swim deeper and deeper and disappear out of sight. He then goes back to the boat, gets on the boat and steers the boat back to shore loving the experience he has just had.

And back on the shore, he goes back to the caravan that he is staying in, he always drives down here in a VW camper van, so he goes back to the camper van he is staying in. He sits down and keeps a journal of his experiences. Not just a journal of the acts that he did and the behaviors, but a journal of his feelings, of how the experience made him feel and

154

what that means to him. And then, after writing his journal he sets up a camp just outside the caravan, just somewhere he can have something to eat on the seashore, a little campfire. And he enjoys the evening setting in, hearing the waves lashing on the shore, on the sand. Birds off in the distance, just sitting there enjoying the evening. Seeing the last of the suns' rays disappear and the stars in the sky. And as the evening draws on, he puts out the campfire, goes back into his camper van and settles down for the night to sleep. And as he drifts comfortably asleep, so he begins to dream and while he begins to dream, he begins to have a dream of himself sitting on a rose, sliding down a rose petal towards the center of the rose and feeling the waxy touch of the petal under his hands as he slides and finding this feeling comfortable and safe and secure. The beautiful scent, the soft feeling of the waxy petal and he knows this dream has something to do with his daily experience. And he goes with the dream. And then he pops through the center of the rose and finds himself sat at a desk in a chateau surrounded by woodland and mountains and finds that his hand is automatically writing as he gazes down at it and sees himself writing something unusual, he sees that he is writing some kind of a story.

He has this sense that he is writing a novel and he gets to a point where he gets drawn into that novel, into a scene where somebody is on a motorbike, going off-road, going around the outside of a mountain, following a mountain pass, following a dirt track. Riding that motorbike higher and higher up into the mountains. And he continues with the scene and there are a few areas where the motorbike skids and then catches the ground again and speeds off even faster and jumps at some areas and the bike is under full control of the motorcyclist. And that motorbike travels all the way to the top of the mountain. And the person on the motorbike is like a treasure hunter. And they are hunting for treasure that is somewhere here on the mountain and the person continues to write and as he continues to write he continues to be absorbed and drawn into this story, drawn into this story as this character discovers a temple high up here in this mountain.

155

And he picks a lock on the door to get into the temple, he walks into the temple and goes from the windy mountain's edge, to silence in the temple. He lights a torch and begins to explore in the temple and while he is exploring in the temple with the torch, so he can hear his footsteps echoing. He searches down one corridor and lights some torches as he goes and then searches down another corridor and then another. Noticing the way that his shadow and the light flickers on the walls, searching corridor after corridor. Until eventually, he comes to a dead end and at that dead end he sees what looks like a trap door on the ground. He prizes open the trap door and climbs down a ladder going deeper and deeper under the temple and as he climbs deeper and deeper under the temple, so he realizes he is climbing deeper and deeper down into the mountain, until eventually he comes out in a cave. And it appears to be a natural cave, it's not a man-made cave. He thinks that maybe the temple was built over the cave on purpose. And he continues to explore this cave. And while he is exploring the cave, he starts to hear dripping water and gradually he starts to hear the distant sound of a waterfall and he continues exploring the cave. And while he is exploring the cave he is looking for some sign of a huge lost diamond, a legendary diamond.

And everything led him to this place and so he continues exploring and while exploring he finds a tunnel from the cave that looks man made and so he follows that tunnel and goes deeper and deeper until it comes out in a room and at the far side of that room is a huge locked door and he picks that lock and enters the room and in the middle of the room is a pedestal with a huge diamond sitting on it, lit up by natural light that seems to be channeled to the center of the room through ice from the outside. And he goes over to the diamond and his plan is to take the diamond and then sell it, but as he reaches the diamond he sees a book. He picks up the book and starts reading and as he starts reading so he learns that this diamond is placed here to bring peace to the land and that there is darkness that will be unleashed if this diamond gets removed. And anyone who discovers this diamond has to look inside themselves and decide what is more important, peace across the land,

156

keeping the darkness at bay, or having the diamond and making lots of money? And he thinks about it. He doesn't know what this darkness is, he can't imagine a real darkness, that would be the thing of legends and myths, so it must be a legend or a myth, it can't be real. The book ends by saying that he is to put his hands on either side of the pedestal where there are two symbols and to close his eyes and that will teach him that everything in this book is true. He thinks to himself that it all sounds ridiculous, but it takes no effort to put your hands on the side of something and to close your eyes for a moment, to prove that it is ridiculous.

So, he puts his hands on either side of the pedestal and he closes his eyes and initially he doesn't feel anything and then he starts feeling a tingling at his hands, that starts in his fingers, or perhaps his palm and eventually starts moving up to his wrists, his arms, his shoulders and in to his body and a warmth, a comfort and he has a sense of a light, a purple light, as if it is given off by the diamond in front of him. He can see it with his eyes closed, he can sense that purple light shining on his face, passing into his head, his body, absorbing into him, this purple light, passing into him, filling him up with this purple light. And he starts to have a feeling of serenity, of peace, of love, of wonder and curiosity, a sense of a connection with the world around him, a sense of what is important. And he finds it a powerful, emotive experience. And then he removes his hands from the pedestal and in a moment the experience passes, and he opens his eyes and he is just there with that pedestal with that diamond and he realizes that the diamond needs to stay where it is and needs to be protected. And he leaves and seals the entrance to that room, and he leaves and seals every entrance behind him and leaves that mountaintop temple and seals the door and then motorbike's back down the mountain with that serene feeling, that learning, that knowledge he gained that will stay with him forever.

And the writer had this feeling that the story was coming closer to an end, as the man found himself with the petals falling down around him, gently floating down to the ground, as he was sat in the middle of these

157

giant rose petals, just falling around him, comfortably, calmly, as he drifted from this dream into a deeper more comfortable, healing, relaxing, sleep.

Conclusion

T hank you for making it through to the end of Bedtime Stories for Adults, let's hope it was informative and able to provide you with all of the tools you need to achieve your goals whatever they may be.

You may have reached the end of the book, but your odyssey into the depths of your imagination is far from over. I encourage you to reread these stories, becoming more and more familiar with their characters and detailed settings.

You are probably familiar with what it's like to reread books or stories and noticing new things when you revisit them. There are simply things you won't notice the first time around.

The joy of reading can be even greater when you come back to stories you have already read, because you aren't only reading to get the story from it anymore. You are reading for the rich detail in the sentences, and for the new perspective you have on the plot and characters since you already know what happens.

Think back to a time when you got really into a book because you so badly wanted to know what happened next in the story. These kinds of books do exceptionally well in the market because they make people always want more. While these kinds of books certainly have their own worth, there is one big problem with them, at least if you are trying to fall asleep.

Since you are reading them as fast as possible just to get the story, you don't get to enjoy the smaller moments that make up the character's journey. All you are doing is reading for information, much like you would a textbook. I'm not denying it can be fun, but it is certainly no way to calm down before bed.

Take the most recent book you have done this with. Ask yourself: did you find that it helped you fall asleep when you read it before bed, or did it just keep you up late because you really wanted to know what happened?

Now, it's actually likely that it helped you get to bed to some extent. That's because stories wrap us up in their own world, so you still let go of yourself and your own stresses for a while when you are reading them, even if you are skipping the smaller details to get to what happens next.

However, it is better to read a book of short stories that are written explicitly to get you to fall asleep. Since you are at the end and you have already enjoyed them, you already know that these stories are still entertaining. They still get your head into its imaginative space and into a world created by words.

But you also know after reading that they were not written for you to simply find out what happens next. Their pacing is nice and steady, so you can enjoy the journey through the story instead of rushing through it to get there as soon as possible.

Therefore, the merit of these stories isn't lost when you read them again. You aren't only reading them to see what happens. You want your mind to create an image given to you by each sentence so you can get your brain to create that image instead of occupying itself with whatever stressful thoughts that might normally keep you up at night. They get you to stay focused on the path you take to get to the end of the story.

The more you immerse yourself in the worlds we sculpted, the easier time you will have letting go of the real world and drifting off to the world of dreams. You can wear the clothes the characters in these stories are wearing instead of wearing your own.

Looking at storytelling from a broader perspective, what the written words is meant to do is give you a new pair of eyes to see the world with. This new pair is always available, but it won't usually occur to you unless you are reading a story.

The world you perceive can be the world of dreams and people who live very far away from you. It can transport you from the day-to-day drudgery and toil and replace it with a great story.

Stories get us to calm down before bed because they activate our default mode network. This is the network of the brain that uses our imaginations and allows us to think more deeply. Using it, you can leave behind the part of your brain that is focused on the present moment, the executive functioning.

Executive functioning does the opposite of what your default mode does. It helps you do things like drive, cook, and do your job. This may be a vital neural network, but many adults struggle to fall asleep because they don't know how to turn off their executive functioning.

The truth is, you can't actually turn it off; you can only disengage it by engaging a different neutral network, the default mode network. The best way to engage that network is by reading stories.

These characters were written to be unique from one another, yet be relatable to any reader, no matter how different they seem to be on paper. I hope you were able to identify with them and their problems, even if you seemed to be a lot different from them on the surface. You are not so different from other people, and that's something that you can learn by reading stories.

It may seem to be a separate goal from falling asleep, but it's really not. You probably found that you have many of the same worries and flaws as the characters in the story, and finding that comparison between you — the real person — and them — the fictional character — will help you bridge the gap between your executive functioning and your default mode network.

Thank you for reading. I hope you were able to fall asleep with their help, and that you liked the stories themselves, too.

Not only were they written for you to have an easier time sleeping, but they were written for you to get your mind on something different from what you usually think about. It's not something that is only useful for getting to bed.

Getting your brain engaged in a fictional story can be good for your stress reduction in general. Short stories serve a variety of purposes and getting to bed is just one if they. You are certain to discover these uses as you continue to read and reread these stories.

Finally, if you found this book useful in any way, a review is always appreciated!

BEDTIME STORIES
FOR KIDS:

26 Children's Stories
To Fall Asleep Fast and Learn Mindfulness,
The best Stories for
Meditation and Relaxed Sleep

Katherine Bennet

Introduction

Bedtime can be a magical time in which you can create memorable moments that will last a lifetime. These experiences are the kind that your children will treasure for the rest of their lives. Moreover, they will hopefully share these stories and traditions with their own children. Indeed, we hope that you have had the chance to make bedtime a time for both fun and relaxation.

In the following chapters, you will find new stories of love and mindfulness, of friendship and kindness, and of togetherness and peace. These are stories that will last for several lifetimes as they are in the following of tradition and heartfulness.

Mindfulness is the key and meditation the rule for having a good life. The stories herein carry with them this theme and have been read by children in some form for many years, and will be read by generations to follow for many more.

As the title suggests, this book contains 17 bedtime short stories for children, best stories for meditation and relaxed. There are so many benefits to reading aloud to your child! Reading aloud to kids prepares them for school success by developing language skills such as proper grammar, the correct arrangement of words, and vocabulary proficiency.

Reading fiction and personal nonfiction, helps a child learn empathy, a crucial social skill to have. When they learn how to express their feelings, and learn the correct terms for them, they are empowered in areas such as conflict resolution, compassion, generosity, and learn how to stand up for themselves and others in appropriate ways.

As you begin or continue on this journey with the kids in your life, take the time to find a place that's comfortable for everyone involved. This

164

location should be free of distraction. Dedicating a usual time in your nighttime routine will help foster the feelings of relaxation. Enjoy these moments! They are fewer and more precious than they seem!

There are lots of books on this subject on the market, thanks again for picking this one! Each effort was made to guarantee it is full of as much useful information as possible; please enjoy it!

CHAPTER 1

Laziness and work

O nce upon a time, there was a very lazy boy. He never picked up his toys; he was always mean and did not understand why he should always tidy up his room after playing and pick up his toys. His mom and dad, who were always unhappy with the fact that the boy is lazy, had to clean up the mess he made. One day, the boy went for a walk with his father and asked him to explain to him why he needed to pick up his toys and why he cannot simply be lazy.

Dad thought about it for a second and then said:

"Let me show you." He called the boy over to a small earthen hillock and showed him how many ants were moving around inside, dragging together various heavy things and arranging their home.

The boy asked him why they do it. The dad replied that even small creatures are constantly working because it is very good and brings them much benefit.

Dad took the boy further, and they came to a large beehive. The boy saw how bees, buzzing and whirling, gather nectar from the flowers, and then carry their prey to their hive. They work such a hard day after day and never get lazy. After all, laziness is very bad, and working allows bees to provide themselves with honey for the winter.

After that, Dad took the boy by the hand and led him to the river. There was a very large dam on the river, which was strengthened every day by beavers. The hard-working beaver went to his dam with a new branch and returned back. Dad showed the dam to the boy and said that the beaver was never lazy, constantly working, and day after day,

166

strengthening his dam. After all, only by working hard, he manages to keep his house underwater.

Dad ended his walk with the words that if all animals work, then people especially should not be lazy. That's why you should always pick up your toys, help your father and mother.

When the boy came home and started playing with his toys in the evening, he remembered about various animals that never get lazy. After playing, he picked up all the things and put them in their places, because if he does not get lazy, then this means that he will help his father and mother.

Seeing that the boy had picked up his toys, his father nodded with a smile, and his mother was very happy. Since that time, they started calling the little boy a little helper because he was never lazy and always helped his parents. For this, he was always praised and spoiled by pleasant surprises because the boy deserved it with his work and the help that he provided to his parents.

CHAPTER 2

Two Elves in the House

Everyone knows about Santa's elves. There's a song about them, stories about them. Little decorations you hang on your tree for them. They get all the credit and all the attention. But what most people don't know is that there are a lot of different elves. Lots of types and kinds that are all over the world! There's tree elf, the river elf, the flower elf, and the moon elf. There's the elf that dances and cares for the bonfires at night. There is the elf that protects the secret places where magic sleeps. There is the wise elf, who tiptoes around the whole world gathering information. There's the wealth elf, who slips under your feet just to pick up loose change or a lost penny. And let's not forget about the music elf, who sing new songs into the ears of the Big Folk. They fill a room with the magic of dance and laughter.

And then there is us. We're the house-elves. You may have heard of us, or maybe not. But whether you know it or not, we're there. It is always helping you Big Folk in any way we can. Not because we must, but because we want to. It makes us happy to see you happy. To see your silly faces smiling all wide when you find something you lost. A toy or a sock, it doesn't matter what. Have you ever got up in the middle of the night and found just what you needed right there in front of you? Have you ever almost dropped something, only for it to land perfectly fine on the ground? What about when you get home after a long day, and the whole house is nice and warm, or it's filled with your favorite smell? Yeah, that's us!

We're the house-elves, and we love to help. Not every elf loves to help, but we house-elves do. We don't help Santa, though. We help you. And

168

that's why I'm writing this letter to you, Big Folk. Because we're sad that you don't know we are there. So, I thought I'd tell you a story. A story of how we, the house elves, helped Santa's elves make a magical Christmas. It's not a long story, don't worry. But it is one of my favorites.

My name is Sniff. Sniff the House Elf. I've lived in my house for over eighty years. I've helped three generations of families that have lived here, but this story is about the first family. They weren't a big family, and they weren't very rich, but that didn't matter to them. Oh no, what mattered to my family was that they were together. They didn't care about money, or who got the biggest present. They cared about getting to laugh and sing on the one day where nobody had to work. Christmas Eve.

That's right; it was Christmas Eve. The Papa came home early with a bundle of goodies in his arms. He worked at the local grocer, so they gave him whatever they couldn't sell at the end of the day. It was Christmas, after all. He had a big block of cheese, a basket of plums, a box of cookies, and a ham just big enough for the four of them to share. Mama came home with a bundle of clothes in her hands. She worked as a seamstress, sewing clothes for rich folk. And because of that, she always had scraps of fabric leftover. And so, whenever she had a free moment away from the loom, she would sew together the spare pieces of fabric. It took a long time, but she finally gathered enough scraps of cloth together to make something nice for everyone in the family.

The two kids, Molly and George, came home early too. They had been running around town all day long, trying to find whatever they could to make the house special for the day. George worked hard at the lumberyard and gathered lots of wood scraps for the fire. That way, they could keep it going all night long. And Molly went all around town, asking store owners if they had any old decorations they didn't need. So, George walked through the door with two big bundles of wood in his arms, and his little sister came in with a pile of garland and some pretty glass balls for the tree.

169

It was a very good Christmas Eve. The dog slept on the rug by the fire, while everyone danced around Christmas Tree. They decked the halls with Molly's decorations, and George made sure to keep the fire nice and hot. The Mama tucked her presents for everyone under the tree in secret, then she and the Papa made a big meal out of the goodies Papa brought home. To anyone else, the tiny Christmas Tree and the lack of presents and the smaller-than-average meal on the table would have been a sad sight. But to my family, it was more than enough because they had each other.

And then, after a night of dancing, singing, laughing, and playing, everyone climbed into bed together for a night of sleep. Santa Claus would be here soon, and they all wanted to be in their bed when he came. What they didn't know is that it was the elves who came first. They needed to make sure everyone was sleeping tight, so Santa could do his work without being seen.

But not everybody was in bed. I, Sniff the House Elf, was up. I'm always up, you see. I needed to ask Santa's elf for a very special favor. I wanted to do something to show the family how much I loved them. But I didn't think I could do it alone. I needed help. And who better to help me with what I wanted to do than Santa's elf? So, when the little green-and-red elf popped up under the Christmas tree, I was waiting.

"Hi, there!" I said to the elf, as nice as I could be.

"AH!" The elf cried, falling on her butt. I didn't think she'd get so scared, or I would have been more careful.

"Oh, I'm sorry! I didn't mean to scare you. My name is Sniff. Sniff the House Elf. Nice to meet you."

"Oh. Just another elf. Well, nice to meet you, Sniff! I'm Maple, one of Santa's elves. What are you doing here? You know it's Christmas Eve, don't you?"

"Yes, yes, I do!"

"Well, you know you aren't supposed to be around on Christmas Eve. We have to do our work tonight."

"Oh, I know that. I do. But I need to ask you for a favor. I want to give my family a special gift. Can you help me?"

"Well, that depends. What's the gift?"

"Come on, and I'll show you."

I climbed down into the hole that led beneath the house. That is where we house-elves live, you see. Under the floorboards, in the walls. Odd places, but we find them cozy and warm. And in my little cubby under the floor, I had a bunch of things I wanted to give my family.

"You see, it's against the House Elf Rules for stuff to just appear the way I want it to. But that's only on most days."

"And today is Christmas." Maple said, knowing where I was heading. "It's magical. So, things can appear, and it wouldn't break your rules, right?"

"That's right! You're one sharp Christmas cookie. Over the years, I've collected a lot of things for my family. I didn't know if I'd ever get the chance to give it to them, but I kept them. Just in case!"

"And now you want me to help you? But what can I do?"

"Well, I have to do a lot. I got all these candles, you see. I want to get them lit and put them around the house. And I carved all these little nutcracker soldiers. I know they aren't as good as the ones you'd make, but-"

"No! Sniff, these are beautiful." Maple took one of my nutcrackers in her tiny hands, turning him over.

"Oh, you really think so? I painted them with wild berries. That's why their coats are all different colors. Some of them are red, and some of them are blue. Some are even purple!"

171

"They're very pretty." The Christmas elf said, smiling at me. She had bright rosy cheeks and short blond hair that touched her shoulders. I thought she was very pretty, too, even though she was a bit bigger than I was.

"Golly, Maple. Thanks so much. I've also got gifts that I found outside."

"You went outside of your house?"

"Yeah! I know it is against the House Elf Rules, but it was for my family. They work so hard; I think they deserve this."

"You really love your family, don't you?"

"Yeah! They're the nicest family I've ever had. I've been to other houses, but this one is the best. They're so sweet to each other. They hardly ever make a mess, and they always laugh or sing together. I want them to know I love them. And since I can't tell them, I figured I'd show them."

"But what if they don't know these are from you?"

"Well, that's okay! They'll know someone loves them very much. And that's all that matters."

"Alright, I've decided. I'll help you." Maple said, nodding her head, making the bells on her hat jingle. "Let's get to business! We don't have much time."

And so, on that Christmas Eve, Maple the Christmas Elf and I worked hard together. House elf and Christmas elf, side by side. We placed the candles on platters around the house and lit them. Now it wasn't just the fire that filled the house with light. The whole house was glowing a soft orange! We took my nutcracker soldiers and put them all over— some on the fireplace and some under the Christmas tree. We set up a little display of them in rows on the dining table and surrounded them with more candles. We took the glass orbs that I had collected and put them on the Christmas tree. They looked so pretty, sparkling in the candlelight. We strung old garland across the ceiling. When it was done,

172

we started to swing from strand to strand, like they were sparkly vines in a Christmas jungle.

"Alright, it's time to put the gifts beneath the tree. So, what did you get them, Sniff?"

"Well, Papa has always wanted to play music. So, I found him this old horn. I've polished it up with oil, so it should play really nicely. And even though Mama makes pretty clothes for everyone else, I know she's always wanted a long gown of her own. So, I got this out of the attic for her. It's old and has a few holes from moths, but I think she can fix them."

"Oh, it's so beautiful, Sniff! So elegant and such a pretty silver color. And the horn! It must have taken you a long time to polish off all the rust and make it shine. What did you get the children?"

"Well, George wants to build things when he becomes a full-sized Big Folk. So, I found him this hammer and screwdriver, and a wood chisel! And Molly wants to explore the world on a boat. So, I found her this fancy hat and old telescope. The hat has some holes, and the telescope needs a new lens. But she's a smart girl. I bet she'll fix it!"

"Oh, Sniff. You know what? Maybe you're half Christmas elf. You've got a real gift for giving gifts." She smiled at me, and I almost started crying happy tears. That was the nicest thing anyone had ever said to me.

"Ah, Maple! Thank you. I couldn't have done this without you. Do you really think that they will like the gifts?"

"I think they will LOVE them."

We smiled at each other, and then we wrapped the gifts up real nice. I was worried I wouldn't be able to wrap them since I didn't have any wrapping paper. But Maple said a good Christmas elf always carries some. And she was the best Christmas elf. And then, once the gifts were all nice and dressed, we put them under the tree together.

173

"Well, that's the last of it. I better get back up to the roof and let Santa know he's good to come on down. It was really nice meeting you, Sniff!"

I couldn't think of anything to say. So, I hugged Maple and squeezed her tight. She was bigger than me, so I could only hug her waist, but she hugged me back.

"Will you come back next Christmas, Maple the Christmas Elf? We can do this again."

"Maybe I will Sniff the House Elf. Maybe I will. Until then, Merry Christmas!"

And then she vanished in a cloud of silver dust. When the next morning came around, the tree had so many presents under it; my family didn't know what to do. George laughed, and Molly screamed. The Mama and the Papa started to cry happy tears when they saw how beautiful the house looked. George really liked seeing all the nutcrackers lined up on the table. Molly started singing a sweet song about decked halls when she saw the garland hanging from the ceiling. I watched through the walls, doing a little dance of my own. I was so happy to be a part of their Christmas!

"Look, Mama! Papa! These presents are different from the rest."

"You're right, Molly. Good eyes." The Papa said, patting his daughter on the head and pulling out the gifts.

"Look, darling. The wrapping is different." Mama said to him, touching his shoulder gently.

"Yes, and there's a note!" George cheered. "Papa, is it from Santa?"

"It is my boy. It says 'Dear Everett Family; it's Santa. I hope you're having a very Merry Christmas. I'm leaving this note with these gifts to tell you a little secret. They're not from me. That's right. They're from someone very special, who loves you very much. You know that I have helper elves. But did you know that you have your own helper elf too?

174

His name is Sniff, and he is a house-elf. He lives with you, though you can't see him. He's the one who did all of this for you__the decorations and nutcrackers, and these presents. He did it to show you all how much he loves you. He's probably there with you right now! Under your feet or maybe in the walls. I just thought you'd like to know that there is someone else in your family, hoping to help you however he can. Merry Christmas! From Santa Claus and Sniff the House Elf.' Well, how about that?"

"We have our own helper elf? Amazing." Molly and George said together.

"That'd explain a lot, wouldn't it, dear?"

"Sure does! Well, wherever you are... Thank you, Sniff!"

And that's the story of how a Christmas elf and a house-elf worked together to make a very special Christmas for one lovely family. So, the next time you find a lost sock or your favorite locket, or come home to your house looking extra clean, be sure to thank your house elf. Because we are there all year round, and we love you. You Big Folk make every day Christmas for us. Thank you.

Sincerely,

Sniff the House Elf

THE END

CHAPTER 3

Once Upon a Time

Once upon a time, far, far away in the animal kingdom, the animals lived together in peace and harmony. They cared for one another, and they took care of the forest they lived in.

Somewhere close to the middle of the forest, there was a very big and fruitful tree. It was a beautiful and strong tree, and it was the biggest tree in the whole forest. It grew near a cool and clear stream; it had several long branches and healthy green leaves.

A lot of birds built their nests and lived in this tree. Some of the animals also built their holes and houses in the tree. They lived in it with their families. Several other animals loved to sit under the big tree, away from the heat from the sun. It was a cool shade on a warm day.

One day, the animals noticed something very strange. The big tree was drying up, and the leaves were beginning to turn brown and fall off. It was also frightening to see the long branches of the tree breaking away.

The birds living in the tree feared that they might lose their homes. They began to wonder where they would move their family too. Many of the trees around were already occupied. The animals living in the big tree were also unhappy because they might start to look for another home if anything happened to the tree.

The other animals who took shelter under the tree were equally sad because the tree was a good shade, especially on sunny days. Sometimes they hold meetings and picnics under the tree. What were they going to do if the tree eventually dried up?!

The animals called everyone, and they held a meeting under the big tree. They discussed how they were going to stop the tree from drying up. The hummingbird came up with a suggestion.

"I think the big tree needs some nutrients," she said. "This is why it is drying up," she added.

"Nutrients?" the rabbit was confused. "Does the big tree eat food as we do?" he asked.

"Yes, of course, the big tree eats too," the hummingbird replied. "But the big tree doesn't eat the kind of food that we eat, silly. It needs a lot of sunlight and water to grow," she said.

"Oh, I see," the rabbit smiled with understanding.

"There is a lot of sunlight," the gazelle said and looked up at the bright sky. "We have more sunny days recently," she added.

"That is true. It has been a while since it rained," the hummingbird said. She had also noticed the change in the weather.

"No wonder the stream is also drying up. There is no rain," the tortoise realized that the big tree needed water from the rain.

"Oh, no! We won't have water to drink if the stream dries up too. We are going to be thirsty. The next stream is far away," the gazelle wailed.

"We need rain. Lots and lots of rain," the hummingbird said to all.

"But, how do we get rain?" the rabbit was confused again.

Everyone was quiet for a while. None of them had the skill or power to make rain.

"I heard that some rain clouds are behind the hill. If we ask them, they might come over and give us rain," said the tortoise.

"But, how do we get to the hill? It is a two days journey," the gazelle complained.

177

"Will the rain clouds agree to follow us?" the rabbit asked.

"If you ask them politely, they will follow you," the tortoise assured them.

"I can fly, so can my friends," the hummingbird said to the gazelle. "We will get to the hill in time," she was optimistic.

"The big tree is drying up so fast, I hope the rain clouds will come soon enough," the rabbit looked up the tree.

"We can only hope for the best," the tortoise breathed out loudly.

"I will call two of my friends. We will go to the hillside immediately," the hummingbird flew away.

"Safe flight!" the tortoise said aloud.

"Please get back soon," the gazelle said to the hummingbird.

"What do we do now?" the rabbit asked.

"We wait and hope for the best," the tortoise said to the rabbit.

The hummingbird, the woodpecker, and the sparrow flew off to the hillside to look for the rain clouds.

"I am hungry," the sparrow said.

"I am thirsty," said the woodpecker.

"So am I, but let's get to the hillside first," the hummingbird said to her friends.

"If I don't eat now, I won't be able to fly another mile," complained the sparrow.

"If I do not drink some water now, I fear I won't be able to flap my wings," the woodpecker grumbled.

The hummingbird sighed heavily. She was aware that she couldn't go to the hillside on her own. She needed the company of her friends. She knew that she would have to give in to their needs until they turned back and returned home.

"Alright, then. Let's look for some food to eat and drink from the river down there," she pointed at a river flowing in a zig-zag motion.

"That's a good idea," said the sparrow, she was very happy that she would get to eat something before they headed up the hill.

"That's a nice suggestion," said the woodpecker, he was greatly relieved that he would get a drink from the river below.

The hummingbird, the sparrow, and the woodpecker flew to a wheat field nearby. They ate until they were full. Then they flew over to the river and took a drink. They were indeed satisfied.

"I need to take a rest. I am very tired," said the sparrow. The food she ate made her feel very sleepy.

"I need to take a nap, I am too full of flying," said the woodpecker. He assumed that he wouldn't be able to go anywhere until he had his siesta.

The hummingbird wasn't happy with her friend's excuses. She was worried about the big tree and their drying stream. They needed rain as soon as possible. But her friends were slowing down their journey.

"We will rest and nap for a few minutes," she said. She hoped that her friends would be ready to continue their journey once they were well-rested.

The woodpecker and the sparrow were happy. They all settled on a nearby tree and napped for a while.

About two hours before sunset, the hummingbird woke up and turned to her friends. She discovered that they were still asleep.

"Wake up, wake up, we need to leave now," she said to them. She hoped that they would get to the hillside in time.

179

The sparrow opened one of her eyes. She didn't feel like going anywhere. She felt like remaining on the tree and sleeping for the rest of the day. "I am still resting. I cannot fly just yet," she flapped her wings and closed her eye.

The woodpecker yawned loudly. He felt more tired than before. He doubted if he would be able to follow the hummingbird to the hillside. "I am not done with my nap. I will be ready in the next hour," he stretched out his wings and started to doze off again.

The hummingbird frowned at her friends. She was not happy with them. If she decided to wait for them, the sun would definitely set before they get to the hill. It would also be too dark to start looking for the rain clouds on the hill.

"We need to leave now. We cannot wait any longer," the hummingbird said to her friends.

The sparrow opened her eyes and regarded her friend. "Why don't you rest a while? We will all go to the hillside soon enough," she closed her eyes and turned away.

The woodpecker yawned again and looked at his friend. "Don't be in such a haste. Take a nap. We will get to the hill before the sunset," he said and turned away.

The hummingbird shook her head. "I cannot stay here with both of you and wait till you are ready to leave. I am worried about the big tree and our stream. I need to get help. I need to leave now," she said to her friends and flew towards the hill.

The sparrow and the woodpecker didn't respond. They were both bent on remaining on that tree.

On her way to the hillside, the weather changed. It grew very, very hot, and a fierce wind began to blow. The hummingbird kept on flying, but soon, the wind blew her off her path. The wind took her in a different direction.

180

Several minutes later, the weather returned to normal. The hummingbird was relieved. She continued her journey as soon as possible.

The hummingbird tried to fight the fierce wind, but soon she gave up. If her friends had come with her, they would have been able to withstand the wind. But she couldn't do it alone.

An hour before the sunset, the hummingbird arrived at the hillside. She saw so many clouds, but she didn't see the rain clouds. Where were they?

"What am I going to do now? I can't find the rain clouds. I hope I am not too late," she was very sad.

"Hello, dear," one of the clouds approached her. He could see her pale face.

"Hi," she responded.

"What are you doing so far away from home?"

"I am looking for the rain clouds," the hummingbird replied.

"Oh! The rain clouds?" the cloud asked.

"Yes, the rain clouds," replied the hummingbird.

"They were here this morning. They went away this afternoon, but they will be back tomorrow morning." said the cloud.

The hummingbird breathed out loudly. She knew that if she and her friends had gotten to the hillside that morning, they would have met the rain clouds.

"Would you like to wait for them?" asked the cloud.

"Yes, Yes, I would. I really need to see them," said the hummingbird.

"Alright, then. Come with me. I will show you a nice spot to spend the night," the cloud drifted away.

"Oh, thank you. You are so kind," the hummingbird flew after the cloud.

The cloud took the hummingbird to a fruitful tree. She found a cozy and empty nest there. She went in and slept off immediately. She was very tired.

The next morning, the hummingbird woke up. She thanked the cloud that gave her a place to spend the night. Then she went in search of the rain clouds. She found them playing at the top of the hill.

"Good morning, rain clouds," said the hummingbird.

"Good morning, hummingbird," they responded.

"I need a very big favor from you," said the hummingbird.

"Let's hear it," the rain clouds said.

"The big tree is drying up. The leaves are falling off. And the branches are breaking away," she said.

"Oh my!"

"What a shame!"

"What a pity."

The rain clouds felt sorry about the condition of the big tree. They knew a lot of animals live in it.

"The big tree needs lots of nutrients. The other animals and I fear that we might lose our homes if it doesn't rain soon," said the hummingbird.

"Oh! what a pity."

"What a shame."

"The big tree does need lots of water and sunlight."

The rain clouds knew how important water was to plants and animals.

"Our stream is also drying up. We might not get water to drink in the coming week," she informed them.

"Oh my!"

The rain clouds felt sorry for the hummingbird and the rest of the animals living close to the tree. They knew that the stream was a source of water for a lot of animals.

"I need a very big favor from you. I need you all to come with me," said the hummingbird.

The rain clouds exchanged a knowing glance. They knew exactly why the hummingbird wanted them to come with her.

"We can't come with you just yet. It isn't the right season," the rain clouds told the hummingbird.

"If you do not come with me, the big tree will die. The animals living in it will lose their homes. The stream will also dry up, and we won't have any water to drink," said the hummingbird.

She hoped that the rain clouds would listen to her and offer to help.

The rain clouds came together and spoke in low tones. They began to discuss what they should do. They knew how important it was to follow the hummingbird back home.

"We will come with you," the rain clouds said to the hummingbird.

"Thank you! Thank you! Thank you!" the hummingbird flew in circles. She was so happy.

The rain clouds followed the hummingbird back home.

On their way, the woodpecker and the sparrow saw them. They were impressed with the hummingbird. They felt bad that they didn't follow her to the hillside to look for the rain clouds.

"We are so, so sorry, hummingbird," the sparrow called out to her.

"We should have listened to you," the woodpecker said.

"It is okay. I am just glad that the rain clouds are coming now with me," the hummingbird said.

When the hummingbird and the rain clouds arrived, the tortoise, the rabbit, the gazelle, and every other animal living close to the stream were very happy when they saw the rain clouds.

Initially, some of them thought the hummingbird wouldn't be able to convince the rain clouds to come to their neighborhood.

But now, they were greatly impressed.

When the rain clouds saw the state of the big tree, they knew that they needed to act immediately. They gathered above the big tree, and soon enough, it began to rain.

It rained and rained and rained for a very long time. The birds and the rest of the animals came out of their houses, and they began to play, dance, and sing in the rain.

The next morning, when the hummingbird woke up, she was glad to see the stream flowing properly, and the big tree was looking very healthy. A lot of animals gathered at the stream. They were drinking, playing, and swimming in the cool and refreshing water.

She also saw several animals sitting under the tree. The sun had risen, and the tree made a very good shade for them.

The hummingbird was very happy because her home was safe, and so were the homes of other animals living in the tree.

CHAPTER 4

Speaking Animales

H ave you ever wondered what it might be like to be able to speak to animals? What if you could understand them and they could understand you? Wouldn't that be cool! Well, you can actually do that right now, without having to even move a single muscle. You really can- In your mind! Your mind is capable of doing many incredible things, including something called Visualization.

To begin your visualization practice, close your eyes. Really, close your eyes (unless you are the one reading this, of course!) To build a very strong visualization, it is usually helpful to the first center yourself and be sure you are giving your brain the very best tools it needs to work with. In this case, that means oxygen, and oxygen means taking some good, deep breaths.

You are going to take some slow, deep breaths now, following along with my instruction: Breath in very slowly, 1 – 2 – 3 – 4. Now breathe out, very slowly, 1 – 2 – 3 – 4. Excellent. Now again very slowly, 1 – 2 – 3 – 4 and breath back out very slowly, 1 – 2 – 3 – 4 very nice. Once more, very slowly in 1 – 2 – 3 – 4 and back out very slowly, 1 – 2 – 3 – 4. Great!

Take a moment to review how you feel. Are you comfy and feeling good? Okay, great.

Imagine yourself, in your mind's eye, standing outside on a sidewalk by a park. You are walking along the sidewalk, feeling the smooth concrete under your feet. It is a lovely fall day, and the air is crisp and cool. You look around you and notice how beautiful the leaves on the trees are as

185

they change their colors. You can see bright and vivid colors of orange, yellow, red, and many colors in between.

A light fall breeze blows through, and some of the leaves from the trees surrounding the park flutter past you as they fly off the trees. You take a long, slow, deep breath in and say "I love Fall!" quietly and under your breath, to yourself as you walk under a tree by the entrance of the park, only to hear a response of, "I would too if it wasn't so much work!"

You are surprised because there is no one here in the park right now! You look all around you, to your left, to your right, behind you and in front of you, and don't see anyone at all, but you know you just heard someone respond. What on earth?

Just then, you hear the voice again, this time saying "up here!" from just above you. You take a tentative step back away from the tree and look up, still not seeing who this voice belongs to. That's when you see a bushy tail twitching back and forth on a branch of the tree and see the dark brown squirrel that is perched there, tail swishing back and forth as it sits and looks out at you.

You laugh out loud at yourself because for a moment there; you thought maybe it was the squirrel! Squirrels can't talk, that would be ridiculous, right? Out loud, you say, "I could've sworn I heard a voice, but all I see is you, Mr. Squirrel! I know you can't talk, so..." as you make a silly expression on your face and turn to go. You stop dead in your tracks when you hear the same small voice say again, "Just because you've never talked to a squirrel doesn't mean you need to be rude about it!"

You slowly turn back around and see the squirrel now leaning back on its hind legs with its little arms crossed across his chest. He is looking right at you! Your eyes wide as saucers, you stammer out "You??? Are you actually talking to me, Mr. Squirrel???"

"Well, yeah! You said you love Fall. I would probably love Fall, too, if I didn't have to spend it preparing so much for winter! I have to gather

186

enough acorns to last me through the winter, so fall is nothing but hard work for me!" the little brown squirrel said animatedly.

You are trying to get over your shock that this furry little animal is talking to you- and you can actually understand it- when you hear another little voice from the other side of the tree.

"Well, it's no walk in the park for us, either. We are getting ready for our long journey south. Trust me, that kind of a flight and your wings get pretty tired!"

"Who is that?!" you ask excitedly as you peer around the tree. You see no one and look back up at the squirrel, who is now pointing up at the branch on the other side of the tree from him. There you see a pair of two beautiful little blue jays, perched carefully together. The two birds raise their wings and wave at you!

"Oh, my goodness! You can talk too!" you stammer out. The birds look at each other and laugh at this. "Well, of course, we do, silly! How else would we communicate?"

"I've never been able to hear you before," you answer. The birds laugh again before answering, "Well, you do! Humans hear birds just fine. Only most of the time, you only hear it as whistles and chirps. Every now and then a human can hear more."

The squirrel is nodding at this. "Yup, usually humans just hear squirrels as chittering and squeaking. Only sometimes can you understand us."

You are so amazed! You had no idea that you would ever be able to communicate with animals! It's like speaking a new language. Animales, maybe! You are so glad that you have had this incredible experience. You are so thankful that these cute little critters decided to talk to you today!

You do not have to leave your new animal friends just yet if you don't want to. You can spend as long as you want here and you can come back anytime, you'd like.

187

You can create anything you want in your mind. Imagine where you want to go and build the picture in your mind. Be sure to imagine how you want it to smell, taste, hear and feel. The more detailed you can make your mental picture, the more you will enjoy being there.

It is all up to you. Perhaps as you drift off to sleep, you may find yourself back in this park, chatting it up in animalese to your new animal friends.

CHAPTER 5

Trip to the Zoo

H ave you been to the zoo before? It's always so fun to see the different exotic animals, isn't it? Well, would you like to go visit the zoo right now? You can do this without moving a single muscle. You really can- In your mind! Your mind is capable of doing many incredible things, including something called Visualization.

To begin your visualization practice, close your eyes. Really, close your eyes (unless you are the one reading this, of course!) To build a very strong visualization, it is usually helpful to the first center yourself and be sure you are giving your brain the very best tools it needs to work with. In this case, that means oxygen, and oxygen means taking some good, deep breaths.

You are going to take some slow, deep breaths now, following along with my instruction: Breath in very slowly, 1 – 2 – 3 – 4. Now breathe out, very slowly, 1 – 2 – 3 – 4. Excellent. Now again very slowly, 1 – 2 – 3 – 4 and breath back out very slowly, 1 – 2 – 3 – 4 very nice. Once more, very slowly in 1 – 2 – 3 – 4 and back out very slowly, 1 – 2 – 3 – 4. Great!

Take a moment to review how you feel. Are you comfy and feeling good? Okay, great.

Now, picture yourself, in your mind's eye, standing in front of a large, black wrought iron gate. This huge gate has the word "Zoo," written in massive letters at the top. You push the gate forward, and it easily opens for you as you walk through.

189

It is a lovely summer day, and the sun is shining. There is a gentle breeze blowing the air that helps to keep you cool. Take a long, deep breath in and notice that it smells like water. You look around, squinting your eyes a bit in the bright sun.

That's when you notice that directly to your left, you see a lovely pond area that is surrounded by a fence. You walk along the concrete path that runs beside the fence, wondering what is in there. You are standing on your tiptoes now as you scan the area, wondering what could possibly be in there when you are suddenly face-to-face with a fuzzy bird face!

Oh! You take a step back with a laugh. You are separated by a chain-link fence, but just about a foot or so away from you is an ostrich, craning its head from side to side, quizzically, as it looks you up and down. Behind the ostrich are more ostriches now in view, approaching the edge of the pond to get a drink.

Their faces are very expressive, and their eyes are wide and interesting as they peer out at you. When they bend down to get a drink in the pond, you giggle at the feathers on their bums as they flounce up and down with every movement.

There is a rock in the middle of the pond that you didn't notice before. It's not very big, but it... Wait, it is getting bigger somehow. Oh, wait! No, it is not getting bigger, but it is moving because it does not really rock at all!

The large gray mound emerges out of the water completely, and you see it is a huge, dark gray hippopotamus! The water cascades down the sides of the hippo, and it stretches its large, blocky head up towards the sun before it opens its wide mouth into a massive yawn! Wow, look at those teeth!

Continuing on the concrete path, you enjoy the feeling of the sun as it warms your skin. Suddenly, there is a shadow overhead, and you realize the path you are on has led you to an entrance of a cave! Interesting!

You enter in tentatively, your eyes needing to adjust from the bright sunshine outside to the darkness of the cave.

Inside, there is a wide-open area in the middle surrounded by walls of glass all around you. On the other side of the glass is something that causes you to exclaim out loud because it almost looks like you are all right in the same space together, but you remember then that you are protected by the glass.

Beautifully majestic lions lounge around on the other side of the glass. You see some lions laying on top of giant rocks, sunning themselves, and some lions down below in the shade, cleaning themselves with their massive tongues just like a housecat!

You are directly in the middle of them and can spin around in circles, watching these beautiful lions as they go about their day. Suddenly some commotion from behind causes you to whip around and see what it is, and you get to see two adorable baby lion cubs as they frolic and play together. The two baby lion cubs approach a lion that is stretched out near them, napping.

The lion cubs look at each other and quickly pounce on the older lion stretched out nearby, and the startled and surprised look on the older lion's face makes you laugh out loud! Those sweet little lion cubs are funny. You are so glad that you are here, and you feel so thankful to be at the zoo.

You love that you get to see these interesting animals, so up close. You do not have to leave this zoo just yet if you don't want to. You can spend as long as you want here and you can come back anytime you'd like.

You can create anything you want in your mind. Imagine where you want to go and build the picture in your mind. Be sure to imagine how you want it to smell, taste, hear and feel. The more detailed you can make your mental picture, the more you will enjoy being there.

191

It is all up to you. Perhaps as you drift off to sleep, you may find yourself back at the zoo, exploring the trails and looking at interesting animals.

CHAPTER 6

Go Kart Race

H ave you ever had the chance to ride in a go-kart before? How about racing a go-kart? Well, don't worry if you never have before because you are going to get a chance to ride in a go-kart race right now without having to move a single muscle. You really can- In your mind! Your mind is capable of doing many incredible things, including something called Visualization.

To begin your visualization practice, close your eyes. Really, close your eyes (unless you are the one reading this, of course!) To build a very strong visualization, it is usually helpful to the first center yourself and be sure you are giving your brain the very best tools it needs to work with. In this case, that means oxygen, and oxygen means taking some good, deep breaths.

You are going to take some slow, deep breaths now, following along with my instruction: Breath in very slowly, $1 - 2 - 3 - 4$. Now breathe out, very slowly, $1 - 2 - 3 - 4$. Excellent. Now again very slowly, $1 - 2 - 3 - 4$ and breath back out very slowly, $1 - 2 - 3 - 4$ very nice. Once more, very slowly in $1 - 2 - 3 - 4$ and back out very slowly, $1 - 2 - 3 - 4$. Great!

Take a moment to review how you feel. Are you comfy and feeling good? Okay, great.

Picture yourself, in your mind's eye, standing outside of a huge race track. It is a beautiful spring day. The sky is bright blue up above you, and the spring sun is gently warming the air.

You look down and see you are dressed in racing gear from head to foot! You have a helmet on, leather racing gloves, and a full-body racing suit. Wow!

Just in front of you is a cherry red go-kart. You climb in, and you are safely strapped in with the seat belt. On either side of your go-kart are large flags with your name written on them! Just right there, for everyone to see, your name!

Now you notice that there are people in bleachers and stands all around the track. They are clapping excitedly, and you see that there is another person climbing into a go-kart right beside you, and they are getting carefully seat belted in. You both look up at each other and give each other the thumbs-up sign.

You are so excited! You are going to get to race go-karts!!! Alright, it looks like you are ready to race. There is a black and white checkered flag that is directly in front of the two go-karts, and it is waving back and forth before you hear a loud popping sound as the black and white kart is raised and you know that means it is time to drive!

You push down with your right foot against the accelerator, and off you go! Your body is pressed back against the seat as your go-kart is speeding up as it travels along the track. You feel great as you fly down the track! The people sitting in the bleachers around you are a blur to you as you are now going so fast you can't really make out details.

You know the other go-kart is nearby, but you have such a fantastic time you don't even really care if you will win or lose, you are just happy to be here racing! The rumble of the engine underneath you is getting stronger the faster you go. You can feel it vibrating throughout your entire body now!

You are vaguely aware of the other go-kart nearby, and you are not really sure is ahead right now. It doesn't seem to even really matter when you are having such a great time racing around this track! You can see something up ahead and in the distance that looks like it might have

194

lights on it. Yes, you can see it now! It is the finish line, and it is lit up with strings of lights that go over and across the entire track.

You are so close! You can still hear the cheering from the crowd around you, but you are zoned in now on the finish line. You know you are getting closer and closer, and you push the gas pedal down completely to the floor of the go-kart as you know you need to really push it in this final stretch.

Your go-kart leaps forward, and you are aware, out of the corner of your eye, of the other go-kart being left behind you as you finally race across the lit-up finish line. You have won the race!

Your go-kart rolls to a stop, and the other go-kart rolls to a stop beside you. You feel exhilarated and happy. You unbuckle and begin to climb out of the go-kart and can see the other driver beside you doing the same. Once you are both out, you reach over and shake hands, telling each other that it was a great race.

The crowd is growing wild and cheering your name! You look around and can see everyone clapping and cheering loudly. You are so proud of the race you won, and you smile broadly as you stand in the sun, arms stretched up and out in triumph. You are so happy and thankful that you have been able to participate in this incredible race!

You do not have to leave this go-kart track just yet if you don't want to. You can spend as long as you want here and you can come back anytime you'd like.

You can create anything you want in your mind. Imagine where you want to go and build the picture in your mind. Be sure to imagine how you want it to smell, taste, hear and feel. The more detailed you can make your mental picture, the more you will enjoy being there.

It is all up to you. Perhaps as you drift off to sleep, you may find yourself back at the track, racing around in your go-kart as the crowds' cheer and call out your name.

CHAPTER 7

Feeding the Horses

Commentato [WU2]: Has only 665 words. Each chapter should have 800-3000 words.

In the middle of fields without many trees sat the Double H Ranch. Keiko had never seen anything like it in real life, but it reminded her of the Western movies her dad liked. He drove their rented car past the gates, and Keiko looked out the window at the cows grazing in one pasture. Across the pasture, a cowboy rode his spotted horse along the fence. A big dog ran beside them. Keiko dreamed about riding a horse just like that!

After they were checked in, they unloaded the luggage from their car. They were staying in a bunkhouse! She and her sister Rumi were sharing a bunk. Rumi was older, and she claimed the top bed. That was okay with Keiko because she was afraid that she would fall out!

"You can climb up and see if you like it," Rumi offered.

"No, thank you!" Keiko said. She was afraid to even climb up the ladder!

The funniest thing was that her parents were sharing a bunk bed, too. They argued over who got the top bunk, and the girls laughed because they knew their parents were just pretending. In the end, their mom took the bottom. Keiko was glad she did. Keiko didn't love staying overnight anywhere but home. She often woke up and forgot where she was at first, and it was scary. This way, with Mom on the bottom bunk, Keiko could go get a hug if she needed it!

They ate a big dinner around a bonfire. While they were eating, cowboys and cowgirls told stories about the land and the people who lived there first. They also told them what to expect the next day. The visitors

196

would help feed the horses before breakfast! Keiko was excited about that!

The next morning, a real rooster crowed right outside their bunkhouse. The family got dressed and went to the barn.

"Good morning!" said the ranch hand. "The horses are hungry, so come into the feed room, and I'll show you what to do!"

Keiko followed her sister. She looked up at the horses in the stalls. They were so big! Even the ponies looked big! They had big heads and big teeth. Keiko wasn't sure this was a good idea!

The ranch hand showed Keiko how to dip a big scoop into the bin of feed. He poured the feed into a can. "This one is for Smoky," he said. "Follow me!"

As soon as they stepped out of the feed room, all the horses started making noises! Several of them whinnied. She could hear one of them stamping its foot! Another was pawing the ground impatiently. She didn't like the sounds! She felt like she was going to get trampled, even though they were all locked in their stalls.

"Don't worry, we're safe," the ranch hand told her. "Here, climb up on this trunk." He helped her stand on top of a big tack trunk that was in the aisle outside of one of the stalls. A dark-gray pony peeked through the bars on the window and made a sound that wasn't as scary as the others she'd just heard.

"He's nickering because he likes you! Here, you see this square, steel door? We're just going to pour the feed right through that."

Keiko was grateful she didn't have to go into the stall with a hungry pony, but her hands were trembling as she pushed the can through the feed door. She heard the feed dump into a trough, and quickly she pulled the can out. "I did it!"

197

After their adventures of the day, it was time to feed the horses again. Keiko was hungry, too! But she listened carefully to the ranch hand's instructions, and this time, she was able to feed Smoky all by herself! That night, she climbed in bed and thought about all she learned. She was so excited to feed Smoky again in the morning.

CHAPTER 8

Lisa Bakes a Cake

Tonight, we are going to enjoy a lovely story about my good friend Lisa, and the cake she baked with her dad!

This cake story is going to be so much fun; I know you will love learning about how to bake a cake with Lisa.

Before we can sink into a lovely story, though, we have to make sure that you are comfortable and relaxed enough to listen!

Make sure you have done your entire beautiful bedtime routine and that you are ready to lay completely still and listen to this story.

If you have not already, get a sip of water, say goodnight to your family, and get cozy in your bed.

Then, we can start with a nice and easy breathing meditation to help you calm your body down so that you can have a great sleep tonight.

Are you ready?

Let's begin with the simple breathing meditation.

For this meditation, I want you to imagine that you are holding a balloon in front of your face.

Can you do that for me?

Great!

Now, let's imagine that you are going to take a nice, deep, slow breath in through your nose, and then you are going to blow out through your mouth as if you were trying to fill the balloon up with air!

199

Starting now, breathe in nice and slowly through your nose, filling your lungs up with air.

Now, breathe out through your mouth as if you are trying to fill a balloon up with air!

Perfect, let's do it again.

Breathe in slowly through your nose, and now breathe out through your mouth to fill up your balloon.

Breathe in slowly, filling your lungs all the way up, and then exhale through your mouth, filling the balloon up with air.

Breathe in slowly, and once again breathe out, filling up the balloon.

One more time, breathe in slowly through your nose, filling your lungs all the way up with air.

Now, breathe out through your mouth, filling your balloon all the way up with air!

Perfect!

Now let's imagine that your balloon full of air floats away into the night sky, leaving you relaxed and ready to enjoy a wonderful story and a good night's sleep.

Goodbye, balloon!

One day, Lisa's dad told her that her mother's birthday was coming up!

Excited, Lisa started planning out what she could do for her mother's birthday.

Lisa was only eight years old, so it was not too easy for her to go to the store and pick out a lovely present to celebrate her mom.

So, she asked her dad to help her pick out a present and to help her bake a cake for her mom.

Of course, her dad said yes, and so in the week before her mother's birthday, Lisa's dad took her to the mall to pick out a present for her mother.

While there, Lisa picked out a beautiful silver necklace that said "mom" on it and had a heart shape around it with three rhinestones in the heart.

Lisa brought it home, wrapped it up, and hid it in her closet so that her mother would not find it before her birthday.

On the day of her mother's birthday, Lisa and her dad took to the kitchen to bake her mother a cake.

They started by gathering all of the supplies they needed.

"What do we need first, dad?" Lisa asked.

"Well, the recipe says that we need flour, sugar, cocoa, baking soda, and salt from the cupboard. Can you get those for us, kiddo?" Lisa's dad asked.

"Absolutely!" Lisa said.

Lisa went to the pantry, opened it up, and grabbed the flour from the bottom shelf, and the sugar, baking soda, and salt from the second shelf.

Then, she looked up and saw that the cocoa was all the way up on the top shelf.

"Can you grab it for me, please, dad?" Lisa asked.

"Great manners, Lisa! Of course, I can." her dad said, grabbing the cocoa off of the top shelf and putting it on the counter.

"What now, dad?" Lisa asked.

"Well, next, we need two eggs, buttermilk, butter, and vanilla." her dad answered.

"Great! I can do that!" Lisa said, opening the fridge to fetch the eggs, buttermilk, and butter.

"Where's the vanilla kept?" she asked, searching high and low for the vanilla.

"Whoops! That's in the cupboard!" her dad grinned, going back to the pantry to grab them the vanilla.

Lisa just giggled and grabbed a mixing bowl out of the cupboard.

"Is that everything?" Lisa asked.

"That is!" her dad smiled.

Lisa went back to the pantry, grabbed the footstool, and placed it by the counter where the mixing bowl was resting.

"Are we ready to get started?" she asked.

"We are! But first, we need the measuring cups and spoons! And a spatula." her dad said, pulling them out of the cupboard.

"Okay, let's get started!" he said.

"First, you need to measure out the flour. Can you measure out one and three-quarter cups of flour?" her dad asked, handing her the measuring cups.

"Absolutely!" Lisa said.

She carefully measured out the flour and dumped it into the mixing bowl.

"Great, now we need two cups of sugar. Can you put two cups of sugar into the bowl?" Lisa's dad asked.

"I sure can." Lisa grinned, adding two cups of sugar to the bowl.

"Now, we need three-quarters of a cup of cocoa powder."

"Okay!" Lisa smiled, adding the cocoa powder to the bowl.

"Can you add one and a half teaspoons of baking soda now, Lisa?" her dad asked, handing her the measuring spoons.

"Of course!" Lisa said, measuring out the baking soda and adding it to the bowl.

"Great, now we need three-quarters of a teaspoon of salt."

"Got it!" Lisa said, adding the salt.

As she added the salt, a little spilled over onto the counter.

"Oops!" Lisa said, looking up at her dad.

"No problem." he smiled, wiping it away with a damp cloth.

"Now what?" Lisa asked.

"Well, it says here that now you need to mix the dry ingredients together."

"Okay!" Lisa answered, using the spatula to mix the flour, sugar, cocoa powder, baking soda, and salt together.

The mixture darkened as the cocoa powder blended in with the other dry ingredients and started to look like the packaged cakes that her grandma sometimes purchased when she did not want to make a cake from scratch.

"Great, that looks good, Lisa. Now, let's add the wet ingredients together. Let's start with the eggs." her dad said, handing her two eggs.

"Can you do it by yourself?" he asked.

"I sure can!" Lisa smiled, carefully cracking the first egg over the side of the mixing bowl.

The side split, and Lisa used her fingers to pry the egg open, revealing a gooey egg white and yolk inside.

She dumped the egg into the bowl, and then placed the eggshell to the side.

She cracked in the next egg, again prying the gooey egg open and letting the egg white and yolk slide into the bowl next to the other egg.

This time, she accidentally got some shell into the bowl.

"Oops! How do I get that out?" Lisa asked.

"Check this out," her dad said, taking half of the empty eggshell and scooping the broken piece out of the batter.

"Woah, how did you do that?" Lisa asked, amazed by how easily her dad pulled the eggshell out.

"Baker's secret." he winked.

"Okay, now let's add the buttermilk, we need one and a half cups of that."

Lisa's dad said, handing her the buttermilk.

Lisa measured out the milk and then poured it into the mixing bowl, watching the thick white milk mix together with the eggs on top of the dry ingredients.

"Done," Lisa said, putting the measuring cup down.

"Great, now let's add the butter. We need to melt it first, so I will do that." her dad said, measuring out half of a cup of butter and placing it in a small pot over medium heat, stirring it regularly to help it melt.

Once the butter was melted, Lisa's dad added it directly to the mixing bowl.

"Now, the vanilla. This is the last ingredient!" he said, handing her the vanilla.

"How much?" she asked.

"One tablespoon." he smiled, handing her the measuring spoons once again.

"Excellent." she grinned, pouring a tablespoon of vanilla into the mixing bowl.

"That's it! Mix it up!" Lisa's dad said.

As she started mixing the bowl, her dad turned on the stove and prepared the cake pans.

Meanwhile, Lisa used the spatula to mix together the ingredients in the bowl.

At first, it seemed like they were not coming together that well, but Lisa kept mixing and mixing.

Soon, all of the ingredients were coming together in a soupy wet mixture.

The batter was fairly wet and thick, but it looked like it would be absolutely delicious once it was done.

When Lisa was satisfied that she had mixed it all the way through, her dad gave it one last mix just to be sure that it was perfect.

Then, they poured the mixture into two separate cake pans, and her dad put them in the hot stove for her.

Lisa was so excited to finish these cakes for her mother that she stayed in the kitchen the whole time they were baking.

She sat on the floor in front of the oven, watching them rise.

At first, it looked like nothing was happening as the cakes simply sat in the oven baking.

Soon, however, the smell of chocolate cake began to fill the house, and the cakes slowly began to rise.

Lisa continued sitting there, watching the entire baking process play out before her very eyes as both of the cake rose and baked all the way through.

When the oven went off, Lisa stood back as her dad pulled the cakes out of the stove and poked a toothpick into the center of them to make sure they were baked all the way through.

"Perfection!" he smiled, showing her the toothpicks were completely clean upon coming out of the cake.

Lisa's grandmother had taught her that this meant the cakes were cooked, but if the toothpick came out dirty with cake batter on it, they needed to be cooked a little longer.

They let the two cakes rest for a few minutes before turning them out onto a drying rack and letting them cool even longer.

Then, they iced the top of one cake and stacked the other cake on top of it.

"A double-decker!" Lisa giggled, looking at the big, delicious chocolate cake they had made for her mother.

They iced the rest of the cake, then covered it in sprinkles and candles for her mother's birthday.

Then, they waited for her mother to get home.

When she did, they lit the candles and showed the cake to her mother, and her mother smiled and blew all of the candles out.

"You made this for me?" her mother asked, scooping Lisa up into a hug.

"Yes, dad and I did!" she answered.

"Here, we got this for you, too!" Lisa said, handing her mother the present they had bought her.

Lisa's mother opened the present and smiled when she saw the necklace.

"It's perfect," she said, hugging Lisa and her dad very close.

"What a perfect birthday." Lisa's mother sighed.

The three of them ate the cake and enjoyed an evening laughing and playing board games together.

When you want to have something in your life, it can be helpful to know how to have the motivation to put the work in.

It might seem easier to go the convenient route and let someone else do all of the work for you, but then you do not get the special feeling of knowing that you did the work yourself.

Doing the work for yourself means that you get to feel proud of the work that you have done, and you get to share the special results with others.

The good feelings you have inside when you accomplish something special is important, and it can help you feel even better.

When you want something in your life but you are struggling to stay motivated to put the work in, remember these important affirmations:

"I can do it."

"I am capable of everything."

"I am great at making things happen."

"If I want it, I can create it."

"I can always try again."

"I am good enough."

"It is more special when I do it myself."

"I can always ask for help."

"Trying counts."

"One step at a time."

CHAPTER 9

The Missing Wallet

This is a story about a missing wallet and how it is always better to do the right thing. One day, Brian was walking down the street. He was on his way home from school. It had been a long day, and Brian had jumped out of his seat as soon as the bell rang at 3:00 PM. All he wanted to do now was to go home, get a snack, and watch some television. Tomorrow was the last day of school, and Brian was very much looking forward to summer break.

As he strolled down the sidewalk, he noticed something out of the corner of his eye. From far away, it looked like a brown square, but as he got closer to inspect, he realized he had found a paper bag. Brian looked around, but there was no one nearby. Brian reached down to pick it up, and he looked inside. Then, his mouth dropped open in shock. The paper bag was full of hundred-dollar bills.

Brian knew this money didn't belong to him, but hundreds of dollars are pretty tempting to adults, let alone a ten-year-old boy that no one was watching. Brian picked up the wallet and shoved it in his bookbag. He told himself that he was going to go straight home and tell his mom, but that is not what happened.

When Brian walked in his front door, he heard his mom call his name. "Brian, come into the kitchen." Brian protectively clutched his bookbag and headed into the kitchen. His mom smiled at him. "Hey Brian, how was your day?" his mom asked cheerfully. Brian should have told his mom then, but he didn't. He knew that was the right thing to do, but something inside kept him from doing it.

Brian's mom handed him a plate of cookies. "I made this new kind of cookie to celebrate that summer is almost here. I call them Lemonades," his mom added. Brian's mom had her very own cookie company, and Brian got to taste them all the new flavors before she put them in her bakery. Normally, Brian felt pretty lucky, but now all he wanted to do was get upstairs and hide his bookbag in the closet.

Brian shoved a cookie in his mouth. "Mmm, tastes good," Brian said, his mouth full of crumbs. His mom laughed. "How about you chew and swallow before you give me your opinion next time," she said. Brian nodded. "Sure thing, Mom," he said, grabbing a couple more cookies and a glass of milk. "I am going up in my room to put my stuff away." His mom smiled. "Ok, dinner is at five. I will let you know when it's getting close." Brian waved at his mom as he headed out of the kitchen and up to his room.

When Brian got upstairs, he walked into his bedroom and kicked his door shut. He set the milk and cookies on his nightstand and threw his book bag on his bed. He sat down and pulled the paper bag out of his bookbag. Brian took a deep breath and blew it out slowly. He had never seen so much money before. He decided to count in. One-hundred-dollar bill after another until he had counted to $5000.00. Brian gulped. He should have told his mom about this right away.

Brian put the money back in his bag and shoved it in his toybox. He knew his mom would never look in there. It was a mess. His mom said she got headaches just looking at his toy box. Brian sat on his bad for the rest of the afternoon, wrestling with his thoughts. He knew what the right thing to do was, but some little part of him really wanted to keep the cash.

Brian jumped when he heard his mom call. "Brian, Dad's home from work. It's time for dinner.", she said. Brian hopped off his bed and headed down to dinner. He wasn't sure how he was going to eat. His stomach felt like it had huge butterflies flapping around it. He knew one thing for sure. Keeping secrets wasn't good for his appetite. Brian knew his mom would ask questions if he skipped dinner so reluctantly, he sat down at the table.

"Hello, Brian. How was school today? Excited for tomorrow?" his dad asked, grinning. Brian was excited, but he couldn't feel it now. He just felt nervous. He put on a smile for his dad, though, and said, "Sure am, Dad. What about you, Kevin?" Brian asked his brother, hoping it would cause his parents to focus on Kevin instead of him.

Kevin wiggled around excitedly in his seat. He was only six. "Yes! Yes! Yes!" he cried. "I can't wait for summer!" Kevin exclaimed. Their dad chuckled. "Okay, buddy calms down. Let's eat." His mom had made fried chicken, green beans, and macaroni and cheese. It was his favorite dinner. Brian silently groaned. Now, he would have to eat a lot. His mom served the food, and the whole family said prayers.

When the prayer was over, Brian took a bite of fried chicken. Normally, he found the chicken delicious, but this time it tasted like sawdust in his mouth. Was he feeling guilty? He started to wonder when he heard his mom say something to his dad. "Ross?" said his mom, "Did you hear about what happened at the children's home this weekend?" his mom asked. The children's home was a place for kids to live when they didn't have a mom and dad. Brian had met the lady that ran the children's home. She was very nice.

Brian's dad turned to his wife and replied, "I didn't. What happened?" he asked. "Well, you remember how they had that big fundraiser last month. We even sent in a donation. Well, Mrs. Smith was running errands, and she planned to deposit the money they made. Somehow, she dropped it. The unfortunate part was that it had $5000.00 in it. She doesn't know how she will buy Christmas gifts for the kids that live with her now. As Brian's dad started to say, "What a shame," Brian turned white as a ghost.

He put his head down and worked on shoving in his food as fast as he possibly could. After dinner, he stood up and asked, "May I be

210

excused?" His mom looked surprised at that, but she told him that he could get up. Brian ran upstairs and sat on his bed. He was scared now. If he didn't turn the money in, then the children at the children's home wouldn't have a Christmas, and if he did turn it in, he would probably get in trouble.

He sat on his bed all evening trying to decide what to do, and he still wasn't sure what he should do when his mom walked in later that evening to say goodnight. His heart must have known, which was better because he just blurted it out without thinking. "Mom, I found the money! I am sorry! I should have given it to you right away!" Brian said, all in a rush. His mom looked confused and sat down next to Brian on the bed.

"Slow down, sweetie. Everything's okay," his mom said gently. "What did you find? What are you talking about?" Brian looked down and slowly got up and removed the paper bag from his closet, and handed the bag to his mom. Like Brian did earlier, his mom's eyes grew wide when she saw what was inside. "Why this must be Mrs. Smith's money," his mom said astonished. "Wherever did you find it?"

"On my way home from school," Brian admitted. "I was going to give it to you, and I knew that was the right thing to do, but for some reason, I just didn't." His mom smiled kindly. "Well, what's important is that you did the right thing, even if it was a little late." His mom took the money and kissed Brian on the top of his head. "I am going to call Mrs. Smith right now. She will be so happy," his mom said.

Brian was so relieved. It felt so good not to be carrying the secret around anymore. Later that evening, he decided he was hungry and ran downstairs to get a cookie. He skidded to a top when he came around the corner into the kitchen. Mrs. Smith was standing there. She must have come by to get her money. "Oh, hello, Brian," Mrs. Smith said, smiling. "Your mom told me about how you found this money and how you happened to turn it in a little bit later than you should."

211

Brian blushed and looked down at the floor, embarrassed. "I forgive
you," she said. "I have a favor to ask, though. I was thinking, we will
have our Christmas party at the children's home and I will need some
help cleaning. I am just betting I can count on you". Brian looked up in
relief. He could definitely do that. "I am happy to help," Brian said.

After Mrs. Smith left, Brian sat alone at the kitchen table, eating one of
the lemonades his mom had baked earlier. It felt good not to have any
more secrets, and Brian vowed not to keep a secret ever again.

CHAPTER 10

Berry Picking Fun

Have you ever been berry picking before? There are so many different kinds of berries out there. In essence, strawberries, raspberries, blueberries, boysenberries, razzle-dazzle berries... well, razzle-dazzle berries are probably not real, but whatever kind of berry you like, picking them is half the fun! What if I told you that you can actually go berry picking right now, without having to move a single muscle? You really can- In your mind! Your mind is capable of doing many incredible things, including something called Visualization.

To begin your visualization practice, close your eyes. Close your eyes (unless you are the one reading this, of course!) To build a very strong visualization, it is usually helpful to the first center yourself and be sure you are giving your brain the very best tools it needs to work with. In this case, that means oxygen, and oxygen means taking some good, deep breaths.

You are going to take some slow, deep breaths now, following along with my instruction: Breath in very slowly, 1 – 2 – 3 – 4. Now breathe out, very slowly, 1 – 2 – 3 – 4. Excellent. Now again very slowly, 1 – 2 – 3 – 4 and breath back out very slowly, 1 – 2 – 3 – 4 very nice. Once more, very slowly in 1 – 2 – 3 – 4 and back out very slowly, 1 – 2 – 3 – 4. Great!

Take a moment to review how you feel. Are you comfy and feeling good? Okay, great.

Imagine yourself, in your mind's eye, in a beautiful clearing in the forest. It is a lovely summer day, and it is still early enough in the day that the weather is not too hot yet. You have been on a lovely hike through this forest, but you are also on a mission! You are looking for an elusive berry species: the razzle-dazzle berry!

The razzle-dazzle berry has just been discovered, and it is very difficult to find. You have been out hiking every day for the last few days looking for this very elusive berry type. You have a field guide that shows what kind of berry you are looking for, and this is very important because you wouldn't want to pick the wrong berry and find out that it is poisonous!

You consult your field guide. The razzle-dazzle berry is bright pink, and it has a property that no other berries have: it sparkles! That's right, razzle-dazzle berries have tiny seeds all over the outside of its fruit, and they reflect whatever light they are in, so when you look at a razzle-dazzle berry, you are dazzled by its sparkle! You review the other information you have about it: it grows on vines in thickets, and it usually grows near running water, so any sort of streams or rivers is usually a good place to start.

Today, you are hopeful because you are heading to a waterfall, and you think there is a good chance you might finally find yourself a razzle-dazzle berry patch! You take a moment to get your bearings, taking a long, deep breath in and smelling the clean, fresh air of the forest. You can hear birds chirping all around you as they sing to each other, but now there is something else that you can also hear; what is that? It sounds like running water!

You continue on your path, much quicker now, following the sound of the water. It isn't long before you stumble across exactly what you've been looking for. It is a waterfall! The waterfall is beautiful, and the spray of the water as it lands in the stream bounces up and into your face, and you smile because it is perfectly refreshing. You are on a mission, however, so you walk along the bank of the stream, hunting for the razzle-dazzle berries that you hope are here.

214

Nothing. You are starting to feel a little worried that perhaps you might not find them when you scramble up and over a particularly large boulder, only to find on the other side something that stops you immediately in your tracks! It is a thicket of sparkling, bright pink berries growing on what appears to be a cluster of vines; you have found the razzle-dazzle berries!

You consult your field guide and check the pictures and the descriptions and make sure that they match with the berries you have found, but the most distinctive part of these berries is impossible to miss, and that is the sparkle! These berries are so bright and sparkly that you almost need sunglasses to come close!

You go to pick your first razzle-dazzle, and you realize that not only is this berry beautiful, but it is also velvety soft, and you gently roll it back and forth between your index finger and your thumb. You decide to give it a little taste, and you pop it into your mouth. It is an explosion of flavor! This berry is sweet and tart and almost effervescent in your mouth- it feels like your mouth is sparkling now, too!

You are so thrilled that you have found the razzle-dazzle berries, and you move along, gently but eagerly plucking the berries from their vines, sampling a berry every few minutes. You are so happy that you found the razzle-dazzle berries, and you feel grateful that you have had this experience.

You do not have to leave the razzle-dazzle berries just yet if you don't want to. You can spend as long as you want here and you can come back anytime you'd like.

You can create anything you want in your mind. Imagine where you want to go and build the picture in your mind. Be sure to imagine how you want it to smell, taste, hear, and feel. The more detailed you can make your mental picture, the more you will enjoy being there.

It is all up to you. Perhaps as you drift off to sleep, you may find yourself back out here beside the waterfall, picking sparkling razzle-dazzle berries.

CHAPTER 11

Zoe Wonders Away

Zoe was preparing for her very first outdoor school weekend. She was reading all the information her Outdoor school leader gave them about where they were going and what they were going to do.

She came across the rules section of the book, and the rule was,

1.   Stay together

Zoe thought since 15 girls were going, that should be easy. Then she saw the 2nd rule,

2.   If you get lost, don't walk around stay where you are, we will find you.

Zoe didn't like the idea of just being lost, but she said, "If I just stay with the group, I won't get lost, and I won't have to have anyone find me."

She finished packing her bags, and she headed out to tell her mom she was ready to go.

"You have everything? Sleeping bag? Warm clothes? Extra socks?" Mother persisted with a long list of everything Zoe should have in her bag.

"Yes, I have EVERYTHING," Zoes replied, rolling her eyes.

They headed to the meeting point. There were already a lot of girls there. They all had their bags lined up by the bus and were wearing nametags. Zoe got out of the car and took her bag to the line and checked in. She was given a nametag and a whistle.

"What's the whistle for?" She asked

"In case you get lost. Rule #2- Stay put. We give you the whistle to blow so we can hear where you are and get to you faster if you get lost." The leader of the outdoor camp said with a smile.

Zoe walked away, looking at her whistle and mumbled under her breath, "I won't need this – I am NOT getting lost!"

The girls loaded up on the bus and waved good-bye to the family standing on the curb waving.

"Ok, our door campers, " the Leader said from the front of the bus, "this is it your outdoor camp weekend, and we are excited you are all here. Please make sure you wear your name badge and whistle at all times. All times girls no exceptions."

They finally arrived at the camp, and everyone piled out of the bus, got their bags and set up their tents. The first evening was quiet with a bonfire, roasting marshmallows and learning who everyone was. They learned what the plan was for in the morning, and they all headed off to bed.

The next day started as early as the sun was up. Breakfast on the open fire and hot cocoa to warm them up from the early morning chill.

"Today girls we are going to be going on an insect adventure," The leader announced. "we will be scouting for and documenting different insects here at the camp. So when you finish breakfast, we can go."

The girls headed out and started looking for insects. Each girl was instructed to locate three different types of insects. They all spread out and began the search. Zoe headed out behind her tent to see what she could find.

Right away, she found two insects she had never seen before. She wrote as much as she could about them and was so excited to find her 3rd. However, she didn't pay attention to the fact that she had walked farther

218

away from the group than anyone else, and now she couldn't see anyone anymore. She looked around and walked back a few steps but still nothing. She began to get scared.

"Oh no, I got lost," She cried. I need to get back to the group. I don't want to be here alone."

She started to head back the way she came. Or so she thought. Nothing looked familiar, and she didn't remember walking by a stream. She was wondering around getting more lost. Just then, she remembered Rule #2- Stay Put. Zoe found a tree to sit under, and she put her backpack on the ground to sit on and wait.

She began to cry and wonder if they would come to find her. She reached into her pocket to get a tissue and pulled out the whistle.

"Oh yes, if I blow the whistle, they will hear where I am and come to get me!' Zoe said excitedly, and she began to blow the whistle as hard as she could.

"Zoeeee!" she heard someone call in the distance. "Zooooeeee!" She started to get excited and blew the whistle more.

Just then, two rangers of the camp came around the corner and found Zoe. She jumped up and hugged them both very hard. She picked up her backpack, and they took her to the rest of the group.

"Zoe, we were so worried about you," another camper said.

"Yeah, we didn't know where you were." Said another

"Remembered Rule 2-Stay put!" She remarked to the group. "That is why you found me- I stayed put."

Zoe felt good that everyone missed her and was glad she was safe. If she had kept walking around, they might have taken a long time to find her, and that would have been scary. She was happy that she remembered rule #2-Stay Put.

CHAPTER 12

A Day at the Pool

S am woke up early on that Saturday morning. He wasn't sure exactly why. Perhaps it was because he had gone to sleep early the night before. His family had gone to a baseball game yesterday, and he had been tired when they returned. But now he was awake, and he couldn't go back to sleep. It was early! He thought. His parents weren't awake yet. Even his baby sister was still asleep.

He walked downstairs and got a bowl of his favorite cereal, Lucky Charms. How glad he was that Mom had remembered to buy it at the store this week! Last week, he'd had to eat oatmeal for breakfast for the whole week! He didn't like oatmeal much.

Sam had just settled down to watch cartoons on TV when he heard the baby crying. After that, the house started to come to life. His mom's tones wafted down the stairs as she sang to the baby. She always sang to Zara as she changed her diaper and dressed her in the morning. Sam's mom was kind of loud, but he didn't mind. Most of the time, he liked it. Sam's dad was quiet, though.

Dad came down the stairs a few minutes later. "You're up early, Sam! Want me to make you some breakfast? Did you already eat your Lucky Charms?"

Sam grinned. His dad knew him well! "Yeah, Dad, I did," he replied.

"I thought maybe we'd go to the pool today," Dad went on.

Sam was instantly excited. The pool! They hadn't been to the pool in ages. "Yeah!" he shouted and ran to put on his bathing suit.

When he came back downstairs, Dad smiled at him. "Calm down, son! We're not leaving quite yet."

Mom came down the stairs next, baby in hand. She set about feeding the baby as she and Dad talked about the family's plans for the day.

Finally, it was time to go. The family piled into their van and headed off down the street to the neighborhood pool.

When they arrived at the pool, Sam saw two boys from school. They weren't his best friends, he thought, but sometimes he hung around with them when he had nothing better to do. Their names were Tim and Christian. He didn't know them very well, but they seemed OK. They saw him right away. "Sam!!!" they shouted. The three boys ran off together.

Sam stared at the sparkling blue water and couldn't wait to get into the pool! He'd been coming to this pool since he was under three years old, so he knew exactly where everything was, and what the most fun things to do were here.

Sam saw his parents walk by and carry Zara through the gate of the splash playground. The splash playground was for babies and toddlers, and it was separated from the big pool by a chain-link fence and gate.

"All together now!" shouted Christian, and the boys lined up and prepared to jump into the pool together. "One... two... three!!!!" shouted Tim, and they all ran and jumped into the pool at the same time, drenching everyone around them with water, including a sweet-looking elderly couple, as well as some teenage girls who were in the pool. Sam noticed this immediately and apologized to everyone. Sam's friends, however, either didn't notice - or didn't care. They continued to behave in a boisterous way, splashing and yelling, not showing respect for anyone else in the pool. The teenage girls glared at the boys and moved to the other side of the pool. The elderly couple pretended to ignore the boys, but Sam noticed that they moved further down the side of the pool towards the deep end, away from the boys.

221

Sam had always been told that he was very mature for his age, and when he hung around with boys like this, he found it easy to believe it was true. He was uninterested in being around this kind of behavior. He began to sort of edge away from the boys, trying to find a way to make an exit and leave them. He knew his parents wouldn't like him being around these boys, either.

Sam looked down in the direction of the snack bar. He must be getting hungry again already, he thought, because the smell of the food was making his stomach water. It was then that he saw Emily. He didn't even recognize her at first without her wheelchair. She was sitting in a white pool chair. Sam noticed that someone was lying in a long chair next to her - maybe her mother? From this far away, Sam couldn't tell. Besides, he had only met her mother one time, so he hardly remembered what she looked like.

Sam decided to go over and say hi. After all, by this time, he was extremely bored with his friends' rude behavior anyway. Emily was more Ralph's friend than his, but nevertheless, he thought she was nice.

Emily didn't see him when he approached her. He thought she looked a bit sad, though. "Hey, Emily!" He said. She brightened up when she recognized him. "Hi, Sam!" He thought she looked thrilled to see him. Her Mom was asleep next to her, so maybe she wanted somebody to hang out with, he thought. For some reason, Sam felt sorry for her. He wondered what it was like to have to stay in a wheelchair all the time. He wanted to ask her, but he knew that would not be polite, so he just sat and waited for her to say something.

Emily was looking longingly at the kids laughing and splashing in the pool. She probably wanted to go in, he thought. So he said, "Do you want to go into the pool? I bet your mom will take you in when she wakes up."

Emily said, "I was just missing how I used to be able to go into the pool by myself."

222

"Oh," said Sam. He wasn't sure exactly what to say, but he felt bad for her. She talked on about it for a few minutes, and so he just stayed quiet and listened. Maybe it would help her only to have someone to listen, he thought. He wished he could make her smile. She looked so much better when she smiled, he thought.

Suddenly, he heard shouting behind him. "Samson!" hollered Christian's voice. He looked over to see Christian and Tim hanging off the side of the pool, hooting at him. They looked unhappy. Sam thought maybe they were mad because he had gone off and left them. "What do you want to hang out with *HER* for?" Tim looked with distaste at the wheelchair under the table, then gave Emily the same look. "Why are you over here talking to a girl!?" Christian asked. Both boys were oblivious to all of the dirty looks they were getting from other people in the pool. Again, Sam wondered if they didn't notice the looks, or if they just didn't *care*.

"Why don't you two go away?" asked Sam crossly. Honestly, he was trying to be nice, but they were getting on his nerves. He wished they would just go somewhere else and leave him - and especially Emily - alone. He didn't like the mean way they were looking at her.

"Are you going to kiss your girlfriend?" Christian asked while Tim erupted into a chorus of "Ooooooh's!" Sam stood up, furious! He was ready to hit the other boy. Luckily, he didn't have to.

"What exactly is going on here!?" Emily's mom had woken up, and she was not happy. She was glaring at the boys. For a moment, she reminded Sam of a protective mother tigress he had seen in a cartoon, and despite all the tension around him, he almost grinned at the thought. Whenever he saw her before, he thought, she had been kind of quiet. She was not like that now.

Her glance moved over to Sam for a moment. She seemed to realize that he was not the problem. Perhaps she remembered that he was Ralph's best friend because she gave a little smile and nodded at him.

223

Then her angry expression returned, and it was directed back to Tim and Christian, who were looking alarmed.

"Where are your parents!?" Emily's mom asked the boys.

Both of them started a little. "They're not here," mumbled Christian. Sam noticed he was now looking a little shamefaced.

"Oh." Emily's mom had a look on her face as though everything was clear to her now. "well, if you don't go away and leave my kid alone, I will be finding out their phone numbers and giving them a call! "

With a few backward glares at Sam, the boys moved away. For the first time, Sam looked at Emily. She looked humiliated. She had been sad before this incident, so now she looked even worse. Sam tried to rack his brain for something nice he could do for her.

"Be right back. I have to go to the bathroom!" He told Emily and her mother. Her mother smiled at him. "Did I hear you standing up to those boys?"

Sam's answer was direct. "Yes. They've been acting rude all day! And I was just tired of it. At school sometimes, they are nice. So, I don't know what's wrong with them today."

Emily's mom shrugged. She frowned. "Yes, sometimes, when boys are away from their parents, they act like that."

"Well, my mom always says I shouldn't get into fights," Sam told her. "So, I'm glad you woke up, 'cause I was getting really mad!"

Emily's mom had one more question. "Aren't you the boy who made the lemonade stand with Sam?"

Emily spoke for the first time. "Yes, Mom. Sam is Ralph's best friend."

Emily's mom wiped something out of her eyes. Was it a tear? Sam wondered. Maybe she just had something in her eye. But when she spoke, her voice sounded a little bit misty. "Well, Sam, you've been a

224

great friend to our family, then. I've never seen Emily so happy as she has been since we moved to this neighborhood.

Sam smiled at her. "I have to go to the bathroom, ma'am," he said again. It was a half-truth, but they did not have to know that yet.

Sam went to the bathroom, but then he headed over to the splash pool to find his parents. He went through the gate and passed tons of screaming, splashing kids who were climbing in and playing around the colorful water playground. He looked for his mother's pink bathing suit and found her on the other side of the pool. His dad appeared to be sleeping in a pool lounge chair, while his mother and Zara were playing at the very edge of the pool. Zara had the blue bucket they had bought for her to play with. Ralph watched as the baby filled it with water, then dumped it out, crowing and clapping after each time, as though it were the funniest thing in the world. He grinned. His baby sister was really cute sometimes!

Then he remembered why he had come. "Mom, can I have some money for ice-cream?" He gave his mom a quick rundown on what had happened. "...and I thought if I gave her an ice-cream, it might cheer her up."

As usual, his mom decided to give him a little lesson from what had occurred. He wanted to roll his eyes, but at least, he figured, this would be a good lesson because he had done something nice this time. He was right.

His mother began, "Ok, Sam, I'm really proud of you. First of all, you went and spent time with someone that probably none of the other kids really wanted to spend time with, because she can't go to the pool. Secondly, you sort of stood up for her - and yourself - when the boys were teasing you both. You know I don't like you fighting, though," she added, as Sam opened his mouth. "I'm glad it didn't get to that! Because there are ways of standing up for yourself without fighting. Anyway, now you're also doing a very nice thing to want to buy her ice - cream to cheer her up! Sam," his mother said, "I am very proud of you today. You are a good kid!"

Sam blushed to the roots of his brown hair. He should be used to his mom by now, he thought, but praise still made him feel shy sometimes - even when it was only his mom giving it.

Sam's mom gave him twenty dollars! He stared at it in shock. She smiled at him. "There's another lesson, Sam. When you do good things, good things will come back to you! So maybe you can buy an ice-cream for both of you, and then you can buy that little LEGO set you've been eyeballing every time we go to the store." Sam laughed. He didn't even know his mother had noticed!

Sam went to the snack bar and bought two giant chocolate-covered ice-cream bars. He went back to where Emily was sitting and handed one to her.

Her face lit up. "I love ice-cream!!!!"

"It seems like girls mostly do," Sam said and started to laugh.

"But boys like it too," Emily protested.

"*Everyone* likes ice-cream!" Emily's Mom chimed in. And they talked and bantered like that for a little bit longer. Then Sam's parents showed up with Zara.

"So nice to meet you. You must be Emily's mom!" bubbled Sam's mother. Emily's mom looked a little overwhelmed by her first. Sam had noticed that his mom had that effect on people sometimes because she never stopped talking. But once you got used to her, though, she was nice. Emily's mom seemed to figure that out because she eventually began to smile and talk to Sam's parents. Sam's mom and Emily's mom made plans to meet one morning for coffee at the neighborhood coffee shop. Then, in a flurry of goodbyes, Sam's family left the pool.

Zara cried on the way home. Sam, who was sitting in the backseat with her, stroked her head. He figured maybe she was tired from the heat. Sometimes the crying got on his nerves, but he was used to it. He just thought, when you have a baby in the house, it's something you have to get used to.

Sam was exhausted. Between the baseball game yesterday and the time at the pool today, he had been in the sun for most of two days. He decided to go to bed early again.

As he went to sleep, he thought again about the day at the pool. He was glad he had sat with Emily at the pool today and also bought her the ice cream. His last thought before he went to sleep was that he liked the feeling he got when he did nice things for people. It made them happy, but it made him feel happy too!

CHAPTER 13

The Sculpture and the Little Boy

A thousand years ago, there was a God named Jupiter. He was down on Earth so that he could be a sculpture and teach the people of the Earth to do better and to adjust, repair, and create many things. He had little comforts as he had lived forever without them and felt that they were more of a detriment than a benefit.

He decided that he would sculpt wood because wood is alive and would quickly learn the lessons that the chisel taught and would carry forward the genetic markers that made good people smile. He decided to sculpt marble because marble could reflect the light that our world offered to all of its children and showed them that they were born good and that they have the choice to follow the pathway of light and not the dark.

He decided to sculpt diamonds because diamond reflects all the colors of the spectrum, and this lets us know that we are responsible for coloring our own lives with the truth and with honesty and nobility. Then, after some deliberation, he decided to sculpt in metal as it was hard and would last a long time and would reflect the sun's rays giving light to those who wrongly chose the dark path.

He thought long and hard about what else he should choose to sculpt and decided to use Terra Cotta because it was light to move about and moldable like the people of the planet. Those who have chosen to do wrong could soon mold themselves into a different form and do the right thing for themselves and others around them.

Then, he decided he needed one more medium with which to sculpt and chose rock. Rock, he thought, will last for a millennium and can show us that our ego can fall away as we are all one. We as humanity are hardbound together as the single sentient species of Earth on the third-density level.

The sculpture walked out upon the Earth to begin and selected a large fallen tree of Oak to begin his work. He was easily able to carry the huge tree back to his work-shed and begin sculpting. In two days, the sculpture had created a form of a man. The form had most of the features of a man but was not yet clear on which man.

Just then, a small boy was walking down the path outside of the sculpture's shed. He noticed the shed and decided to enter it. When he walked in, he was moved by the sculptures work in wood. He asked the sculpture, "why are you working today in wood, and who is this form of a man?"

The sculpture thought for a moment and then said, "I used wood on this particular sculpture for a number of reasons. You, child, have the power to know the answer to your question if you will just walk the high road and continue with the peace and the love that you were born with such a short time ago. Know that this is only made from wood but that it is what made you ask your question of me. That alone tells me that you are indeed on the high road and still carry the love that you were born under. I know that you have been aware of living a mindful life, and you have been meditating. Am I not correct?" the sculpture asked.

"Yes. It's true that my parents are very good and noble people and have taught me many things in my short life. They showed me mindfulness and how it worked and why it is so important for all of us to practice it, and they did this in the first two years of my life." The boy said and then continued, "And you are also correct that I do meditate every day as this keeps me true and stays my direction through my young life."

The sculpture was pleased to hear this and told the boy so. He then invited him to join him in drinking some water and having some food to eat together. "You and I are a family of a different sort. This time

together for families is so very important. I know your family has most
likely spoken of this to you, but I want to say it to you anyway. Family
and the family tradition is the most sacred thing for us to do here on
Earth. So many people do not seem to know this, so perhaps I could
ask you to spread my message of the family to all those you might come
in contact with." The sculpture suggested to the boy. "Thank you for
the food and water kind, sir, and I give you my word in honor that I
shall spread the word to all I meet and know that family is the most
important thing." The boy said.

A few days had passed, and the sculpture finished his wooden form, and
it now resembled a man with a long beard, sitting on an old sea chest
and holding a large three-pronged pitchfork. The sculpture then
dropped to his knees and prayed unto the wooden form and asked that
it take to life. The form suddenly creaked, and the arms moved. Then
the head turned, and the form of the man of wood stood up was over
nine feet tall. He looked down upon the sculpture and said, "I am
Neptune. I am the God of the seas, and I thank you for giving me life.
I must go now and care for all the sea creatures and the people who
venture out over the depths in boats." Neptune then trod his mighty
feet over the shed floor, making the simply wooden walls shake and
seem, for the moment, unsteady. Out the door, he walked and away
from the sculpture.

The next morning, the sculpture decided to sculpt in marble, so walked
a long way to the quarry, where the marble of the planet could be found.
He located a large square block of marble and had no trouble at all,
bringing it back with him to his meager work-shed. When he arrived at
his shed, he set the marble block up on its small end and began to work.
He chipped away here and there until the marble began to appear in the
form of a man. Then, the sculpture stepped back and looked up at what
he had created. Just then, the same small boy was passing by again and
decided to stop and say hello to his new friend, the sculpture. "Hello,"
he called out as he came up the pathway to the front door of the shed.

Why hello there, young man. This is good timing for I was about to take some lunch, and it would be wonderful if you would be so good as to join me?" he said with an inviting smile and a wave in towards his lunch table. "I would indeed love that, and thank you for the invitation kind, sir." The boy said, smiling back at the sculpture. But then he turned and noticed the marble statue of the form of a man and asked, "Why have you sculpted this form in marble, and who is this man you have created?" The sculpture only smiled this time and gave the boy some food that he had previously prepared for his lunch.

"Let us eat and drink water together once again, and I will tell you all there is to tell about this new work I have done." The sculpture said, taking a spoon to his soup. "Come now, young man, eat your soup as I am doing here, and you shall be strong like me for twenty lifetimes." He told the boy. When they were done, they both sat together, gazing up at the marble statue which the sculpture had made. Then the artist spoke again. "This man is called Pluto. He is the God of the underworld. He is the God of wealth and the lord of all that is metallic. He rules over all the riches that lie in wait beneath the Earth." Then, the boy turned to the sculpture and asked, "but why did you create this form in marble of such a man?"

The sculpture looked down at the boy and smiled again, saying, "That is a most astute question, young man. You are perhaps, and you and old soul have wisdom beyond your years." Then they both stopped talking and just stared up at the huge marble form of a man. Then, the sculpture cleared his throat and began to speak once again. "We need Pluto, so we do not get caught up in our own egos and think only of ourselves. We must always think of others who are around us and be sure to prevent any arguments or fighting and use our hearts to send out only love and loving emotions." The sculpture said with a passionate tone. By the time he was done saying these words, he was standing as he had much passion for this subject. The boy was very impressed by the mannerism of the sculpture, which he was beginning to see as a very great man.

231

Then the boy stood as well and looked up into the great sculpture's eyes and said, "I must be getting home now as my parents may become worried about me." The sculpture turned toward the boy as he stood at the entrance to the shed getting ready to leave and said, "Will you give your word to tell everyone you know and may come to meet that the true measure of a man is not by anything more than how he helped those around him. By what he gave of his soul and that he taught others to hold onto their free will and how he showed them to fight for their freedoms and never allow anyone to take from them their selfness?" the sculpture finished. "I will do that always, oh great sculpture. I do give my word to pass this knowledge to all who I may meet along the pathways that I may walk. "

A few hours after the boy had left, the sculpture finished sculpting the marble form and dropped down onto his knees and began to pray. He prayed for the marble statue to come to life and soon heard a strange grating sound. When he looked up into the eyes of the great marble statue, it looked back down at him and moved its arms, then its legs and feet. The great statue jumped down from the sculptures table and walked over to the shed door and then turned to face the sculpture. "I am Pluto, God of the Underworld, and I thank you for giving me life. I must go now as there is much work to be done with the people of the Earth. And with that, the huge man of marble trudged out of the sculptures shed, shaking the walls once again as he headed out down the pathway.

A week past and the sculpture rested and thought about what to do next. Then he got an idea. "People need color and happiness in their lives, and I will help them with that." He mused. The following morning the sculpture walked out and went down the pathway that led through the forest and into the valleys beyond. When he got there, he sought out the diamond mines. Several friendly people who he met along the path told him how to get there, and he finally found the mine.

He selected a huge diamond block and easily carried it back down the pathway, back through the forest and up the hill to his work-shed.

232

There, he began to sculpt the diamond block. He chiselled away and worked long into that night, through the next day and into the next night. Then, when he looked up into the eyes of his newest creation, he knew he was done.

The next morning, his little friend, the young boy came up the pathway calling out to him as he walked. "Mr. Sculpture, are you home today?" the boy called. The sculpture went to the doorway and waved the boy to come in, saying, "Hello there, young man, it is very good to see you and again, great timing. I am just about to have a meal and drink some water. You should join me." He told the boy. The sculpture and the young boy enjoyed their food and drank water together once again. When they were done with the meal, the boy turned to look at the new project the sculpture had created and asked. "so, who do we have here oh mighty sculpture?" The artisan looked at the boy, and then up at the statue of diamonds glistening in the morning sun as it shone down through the shed window.

"Why have you created this massive man, and why did you use diamond this time pray tell sir?" the boy asked once again. "This is Apollo. He is the God of Sun, Music, and Prophesy. Apollo will show our people that they have other things that they can do with their lives, such as play and instrument and sing. He will also show them that they should pray for the power of the sun and its life-giving properties. Without the sun, none of us would be alive on this beautiful planet. He will show them wisdom and direction that will keep them free, and in freedom, he will show them unity for unity is the greatest power in the universe, the sculpture proclaimed.

Soon the boy told the sculpture that it was time for him to go again and stood up to bid him farewell for the time being. They said their goodbyes, and the sculpture watched as the boy slowly made his way down the path and around the corner and out of sight.

Then, the sculpture heard a sharp cracking sound and looked up at his newest creation. Apollo was beginning to move as the others before him had done. First, he moved his head around to look straight at the sculpture, and then his hands and finally his legs and feet. He jumped down off of the sculptures table and walked over to face his creator. "I am Apollo." He stated boldly. "I am here to see to it that the people of the planet are in unity and can express their creative passions. I must go now." He passed out through the shed door and walked off down the pathway towards the town.

After Apollo left, the sculpture went to bed and slept for two full days, for he was exhausted after all of his sculpturings. When he awakened, he decided to create his next project out of metal as the metal was strong and would last a very long time indeed. He readied himself and then went into town to the blacksmith's shop. The blacksmith welcomed him, and they shared some food and drank some water together. The sculpture told the blacksmith what he needed, and the blacksmith said, "I have just what you need in the back of my shop." The sculpture thanked the man and then had no trouble at all, carrying the huge block of metal back to his shed.

He then got right to work sculpting the great block of metal into the shape of a man. Before long, the sculpture finished his work and then sat down across the room from it so that he could stare up at it and think. Then once again, the boy just happened to be walking past the shed and looked in. When he saw the great metal man up on the sculptures table, he couldn't help himself and entered the shed saying hello to the artisan and looking straight up into the eyes of the new metal man. "Who is this big metal man, and why have you created him," he asked yet once again.

"I am happy that you are visiting me today and would like to tell you about this one." He told the boy. "This is Saturn! He is the God of agriculture." He said. "Saturn is here to help the people of our small blue planet grow food and show others how to grow their own crops for this is how we must eat. Of the land and from the Earth. This is the proper way for us to share our meals." The sculpture told the boy. "That is a very good thing to do." The boy said, "I know that because this is what

234

my parents have always done, we have a farm and raise corn, carrots, lettuce, and other vegetables." He told the sculpture.

"I am happy to hear about your family farm, but would you promise to tell your friends and those you may meet that growing our own food is our way and that it is the proper thing to do. Our planet shall always provide food for all of her children." The sculpture said to the boy.

The boy then left the sculptures shed and went about the town telling everyone he met about how having mindfulness, how meditating, and how being kind to each other was the right thing to do. He also told them that arguing and fighting was not the right thing to do and that all disputes, should they ever arise, can be settled through gentle conversation and agreeing on the common ground we each share. After all, we are one human species on Earth, and we must get along and never fight among ourselves.

Then, one day, the boy decided that since he had learned much from the sculpture, he would like to go up on the hill and visit one more time to thank the sculpture for teaching him about how to be a man. He walked up the pathway to where the sculptures shed was, and to his surprise, instead of the shed where it had always been, where he had visited so many times, there was an open field with colorful flowers of reds, blues, and violets growing everywhere he looked.

He took this as an omen that the sculpture's work was done here. The boy never spoke of the sculpture and never told anyone of his visits to the work-shed where he had witnessed the creation of so many Gods who all did good work for him and his fellow humans. He decided to dedicate his life to doing all the good work that the sculpture had taught him. In the years that followed, the boy became a teacher and made this his career and daily life. He was fulfilled each day, knowing that he was carrying on the work of the great man on the hill.

CHAPTER 14

No diligence, no price

In the forest, once lived a hamster and a squirrel. The hamster was always very diligent and did all his duties immediately. The squirrel, on the other hand, was very lazy. It would rather enjoy life; without all the annoying tasks that you had to do as a squirrel.

Every autumn, the animals began to gather supplies for hibernation. Squirrels, hamsters, mice and bears retreated to a cozy hideaway in winter to sleep a lot. Only when they got hungry did they wake up to eat. And there had to be something to eat.

So squirrels, hamsters, mice and bears gathered as much food as they could find and hid them in various places, in tree caves, empty bird nests, in the ground or even under stones. They collected more than they needed. Because it could be that other animals found the hidden food and - unknowingly - took the food of another. Or you forgot many a hiding place. That could happen - there were many.

So the hamster collected as much as he could. But the squirrel was lazy. He did not feel like collecting every day. It preferred to play by the stream or lay in the grass. When winter came, the squirrel realized that it was quite late and began to gather. Of course, time was not enough, and the squirrel was very worried.

It asked the hamster if he would share. The hamster said, "You could have collected enough yourself! Why didn't you do that? "The squirrel, however, had no excuse and replied," I had so much else to do. That's why I did not make it. Please, dear hamster, you have more than you need. Or should I starve to death? "

"All right," said the hamster, sharing his supplies with the squirrel. The squirrel was happy and thought, "Such a stupid hamster. That was easy. I'll do it again next year! "

When the next autumn came, the hamster again diligently collected food for hibernation. But what was that? The hamster saw the squirrel lying in the grass and dreaming. "What are you doing there? Why do not you collect anything? "Asked the hamster. The squirrel was startled but again was not excused: "Did you scare me, hamster. I'm just taking a break because I've collected so much, "it said.

When the winter came, the squirrel had not collected a nut, not a mushroom, not a cone or seed. With a single nut in his hands, the squirrel went to the hamster and said: "Come on, dear hamster, my whole food was stolen! Only this nut was left to me. What am I doing now? Surely you have more than you need, right? "The hamster shook his head." You have nothing? "He asked. The squirrel replied, "Not a nut, not a mushroom, not a cone or a seed."

The hamster said, "I did not find so much myself this year that it would do for two." The squirrel became angry: "You have not found enough for two? Why did not you say anything before? That's pretty mean of you hamster - do you know that? Had I known that, I would have collected myself! "

Then the hamster listened: "You have not collected?" The squirrel swallowed when it noticed that it had revealed itself: "Well, well. I had a lot to do, and then there was little time. "The hamster, however, now realized what he was talking to the squirrel:" That means you lied to me last year. And this year, you just wanted to make it easy for you. I understand that! "Said the hamster angrily.

"But do you really want to starve me?" Asked the squirrel. The hamster shook his head: "No, I will not let you starve to death. I'll give you enough that you do not starve. However, it will be too little to get full.

237

I hope your growling stomach will open your eyes over the winter! "Said the hamster, giving the squirrel a small portion of his supplies.

The squirrel was angry with the hamster and did not seek the blame on himself. It thought, "This means hamster. Had he told me early enough that he did not have that much, I could have collected something! That's all his fault! "Yes, the squirrel was so upset with himself that it was hard to admit that it had made a mistake.

However, the longer the squirrel was in hibernation, and the stomach rumbled, the clearer it became to him that it was all to blame. It had to admit that it had made a mistake. Only then could the squirrel make it better for the next hibernation.

The next autumn, the squirrel gathered day one day. It ran quickly back and forth and collected more of everything. When winter came, the hamster went to apologize. The hamster was very happy about the squirrel's insight!

The squirrel offered the hamster some of his supplies as an excuse. But the hamster had enough supplies this year and said, "I was able to collect enough this year - thank you very much. But other animals may not have been so lucky. They would be very happy if you gave them some of your supplies. "

"That's how we do it!" Said the squirrel and gave some of his supplies to all the animals that did not have that much. The other animals were happy and thanked. But the squirrel said, "I never thought I would say that - but you can thank the hamster. He gave me a lesson that I will not forget all my life. "And so the animals thanked the squirrel and the hamster. Since then, all are the biggest friends and help each other - wherever they can!

CHAPTER 15

Bessie's Ball

Along time ago, a little girl named Bessie lived in a pretty cottage with her father. It was just her and her father. Years before, her mother had died. It happened when Bessie was very little. Bessie didn't remember much about her mother, but she did remember that she was very beautiful and very kind. One day, Bessie's father decided that there needed to be a woman in the house for Bessie to learn womanly things from. So, he decided that he was going to get married and went out into the world to find a wife who could also be a stepmother to Bessie.

After a few weeks of trying, Bessie's dad found a woman that he wanted to marry. He brought this woman home to meet Bessie. Bessie was a good sport and decided that she would do her best to like her new stepmother. What she didn't know was that her new stepmother came with two stepsisters. Bessie had never had stepsisters before, and she wasn't sure what it would be like, but she decided that she would give it a try.

Her stepsisters were named Kelly and Nelly. Kelly and Nelly looked very fancy. They had their hair done up in great big curls with ribbons. They also were wearing dresses in the latest fashion. Bessie felt underdressed standing next to them, and she got the feeling they Kelly and Nelly did not think that her dress was worth wearing. Her stepmother seemed nice, and Bessie hoped that they would hall get along.

Not too long after her father remarried, he began to get very sick. After a few weeks of being ill, her father died. Bassi was heartbroken. She couldn't believe that her father had died and left her alone in this world.

239

She did have her stepmother and stepsisters, though, and she decided that they would be enough and that the four of them could be a family. Unfortunately, her stepmother had other ideas.

After the funeral, her stepmother came into her room and told her that since her room was the biggest in the house, it now belonged to Nelly and Kelly. She told Bessie that she would have to live upstairs in the attic. Bessie couldn't believe that she would have to give up her room, but she didn't mind being upstairs because that was where her mother's things were stored.

The next day, her stepmother told her that she was going to be in charge of all the chores. She was going to have to do the sweeping, the mopping, the cooking, the cleaning, and anything else that her stepmother and stepsisters needed to be done. Bessie didn't mind doing hard work. She liked to help other people, but why was Bessie the only one that had to do it?

This went on for several weeks. Bessie did all of the work and didn't understand why her stepmother was being so cruel to her. Bessie wasn't allowed to eat dinner with them; she had to eat alone in the kitchen. She wasn't allowed to hang out with them, so she was all alone all of the time. She did have a dog, but her stepmother kicked the dog outside, and Bessie never had time to see him. One day, after weeks of cleaning, Bessie's stepsisters came into the room. Bessie was covered in dirt, so her stepsisters decided to call her Messy Bessie. Bessie did not like the nickname, but they thought it was hilarious. It was always "Messy Bessie, go fix my dress", "Messy Bessie, go clean my room," Messy Bessie, bring me a cookie." Bessie was not happy at all

One day, a messenger came to the house with an invitation to a ball. A ball is a huge party where everybody gets together to eat and dance. Bessie was thrilled! She was so excited about being able to go to the ball. The invitation said all eligible ladies needed to come to the ball because the prince was looking for a wife. Bessie wasn't interested in being the wife to anybody, but she was interested in going to the ball.

Unfortunately, her stepmother gave her a gigantic list of chores and told her if she didn't get them done, she was not going anywhere.

The day of the ball, Bessie worked so hard that she got all of her chores done and then went upstairs to the attic. She opened up a chest that held her mother's clothes and picked out a beautiful pink dress. She was going to wear her mother's dress to the ball. She got ready, and she was simply gorgeous. Her long, blonde curls cascaded down her back. She looked a lot like her mother.

When she got downstairs, she told her stepmother that she was ready to go, but her stepmother "accidentally" knocked into her, then her stepsisters "accidentally" tore her dress. Bessie was in tears; she knew this was no accident. They were keeping her from going to the ball. All three of them giggled as they walked out to their car. They left Bessie crying on the front steps as they drove away.

She sat on the steps, feeling sorry for herself. Suddenly, a bright light appeared in the yard with a POOF, and a fairy appeared on her porch. The fairy wore a stunning white dress. She had silver hair, and she was very beautiful. She was also very small and flew over to Bessie.

Bessie asked, "Why are you here? what do you need with me?" The fairy said, "I am your Fairy Godmother, and I am here to help you go to the ball. There's something special coming for you at the ball, and I'm going to make sure that you can get there." With a flick of her wand, Bessie's torn dress was transformed into a beautiful golden gown. It was covered in sequins, and she had diamonds throughout her hair. She looked just like a princess. Her fairy godmother said, "There, look at that! You are going to be the belle of the ball.

Bessie asked, "But fairy godmother, won't my stepmother and stepsisters see me? I will be in so much trouble, and she is sure to give me more chores." Her fairy godmother smiled, "Do not worry, Bessie. My magic will protect you from their eyes. They can see you, but they will not recognize you." Bessie was very relieved.

Bessie told her fairy godmother that she didn't have the means to get to the ball. Her fairy godmother said, "Look outside! I have a brand-new car for you. It's a limousine, and someone will drive you to the ball. You will go there in style." The limousine was long and white. Bessie had only dreamt of riding in such a special car.

Bessie was so happy that she threw her arms around her fairy godmother and gave her a great big kiss right on her forehead. Then she ran and hopped in the car. All of a sudden, her fairy godmother yelled, "Wait! Wait! We need to give you some special shoes!" As Bessie watched, her fairy godmother flicked her wrist again, and suddenly, Bessie was wearing the most beautiful glass slippers. They fit perfectly.

Her fairy godmother said, "Just make sure you're back by midnight because at midnight, your clothes change back to the way they were." Bessie promised that she would be home by midnight. Bessie thanked her fairy godmother and hopped in the car. Bessie watched excitedly out the window as her driver took her to the ball. She felt like a princess living in a fairy tale.

When Bessie arrived at the ball, she walked up the front staircase. It led to the big mansion that the king, queen, and prince lived in. She walked in the front door and stepped inside. All of the guests stopped to look at her. Bessie was the most beautiful girl at the ball. Her long hair shimmered from the diamond hair clips. Her gold gown fit perfectly, and her glass shoes made all the difference. People could tell that she was the kindest and most beautiful girl in the entire kingdom.

The prince was sure to notice. He noticed very quickly. He walked straight to Bessie and asked her to dance. Bessie happily accepted the prince's offer. The two danced for hours, but before longing, it was almost midnight. Bessie had to go back home. She promised the prince that she would see him again, although she didn't know how she would do it.

She ran down the steps out of the house and hopped in her car. Before she got back home, her dress turned back into tears, but her glass slipper did not disappear. Bessie realized one of her shoes had fallen off as she ran down the steps. She wondered if the prince would see it.

The next morning, Bessie went about doing her chores with a smile on her face. "What are you smiling about?" asked Nelly. "Yeah, you didn't even go to the ball," said Kelly. Bessie did her best to keep a straight face. "How was the ball? Did you meet the prince?" Bessie asked. Nelly and Kelly both frowned. "No! We didn't meet the prince! Some girl, with diamonds in her hair and a flowing gown, took all of his attention." Bessie smiled. "Oh my," she said. "How terrible for you." Nelly and Kelly just glared at Bessie, and Bessie went about her day.

Later that evening, Bessie was cooking dinner when she heard a knock on the door. She walked to the door and opened it. Much to her surprise, there on her porch was the prince's errand boy. He handed her a note. It read…" All women come to the town square to try on a glass slipper." Bessie fainted.

When she woke a moment later, the errand boy was looking worried. She apologized for scaring him, took the note, and shut the door. Bessie couldn't believe what she had read. The prince was looking for her. Reluctantly, Bessie handed the note over to her stepmother, who told her daughters to hurry up and get ready. Bessie asked her stepmother if she could go to. Her stepmother looked suspiciously at her.

"No! You didn't go to the ball. Why ever would you need to go?" Bessie looked so upset, and her stepmother grew even more suspicious. She yelled for her girls to hurry up, and the three of them left in a flurry. Her evil stepmother locked Bessie inside her house. Bessie sat down on the ground and began to cry.

A moment later, Bessie felt a tap on her shoulder. She jumped and looked up in surprise. It was her fairy godmother! "Why are you crying, Bessie?" her fairy godmother asked. "Don't you know by now that I

243

always look out for you? I told you the ball would bring something amazing to you. You just have to believe." With a swish of her wrist, the fairy godmother transformed Bessie's old dress into a beautiful pink dress. "It looks just like my mom's dress!" Bessie exclaimed. The fairy godmother smiled. "I knew your mother. I was her fairy godmother too."

The fairy godmother proofed some pink, satin shoes onto Bessie's feet. Bessie grabbed her glass slipper and headed out to the car, waiting for her outside. Bessie hopped in, and the driver sped off, getting her to the prince. Bessie clutched the glass slipper. Could this be happening? Was the prince looking for her? Could he love her? Bessie knew she had fallen in love with the prince last night.

Bessie finally got to her destination, and she saw a line of girls wrapped around the prince's errand boy. No one could fit into her glass slipper. Bessie had always had small feet. She crept closer and watched Nelly and Kelly try on the shoe. They both had gigantic feet, so obviously, the shoe did not fit. Bessie began to laugh out loud, and that is when her stepmother noticed her. "This girl does not belong! She was not at the ball!", her stepmother screamed. Bessie gathered up her courage and shot back, "Yes, I did! I have the second glass shoe!" The errand boy's eyes grew wide, and out of the crowd stepped the prince. He had been hiding in plain sight the whole time.

"Beautiful Bessie," called the prince. "May I help you with your shoes?" Bessie blushed and walked to where the prince stood. "Anytime," she said, and she kissed him. He knelt to put on her glass shoes, and then he pulled out a ring. "Will you marry me, Bessie?" he asked. Bessie grinned. "Yes! Yes! A thousand times, yes!" she cried. The prince slid the ring on her finger, and she kissed him again.

Betsy's dreams had come true. The look on her evil stepmother and stepsisters' faces was priceless. Bessie completely ignored them. The errand boy went to her old house and gathered her possessions. Bessie and the prince went with him so that she could say goodbye to her

244

home, and then she turned and walked into the prince's arms. She walked into her future and left the past behind.

CHAPTER 16

Bedtime Story

It was late evening, and little Vincent was ready to go to bed. Every night, after dinner, he and his grandmother would sit in his room, reading all kinds of stories. This night wasn't any different. Grandma tucked in Vincent, and he lay down as his grandma was setting up her chair. She sat next to him. "What would we read, Vincent?" grandma asked. "Should we go with the one we read last week. About cars?"

Vincent thought about what to say. "We've been through every book there is. Could we improvise this time?" he asked. Vincent's grandma thought about his proposition and asked, "OK. Are you ready for this one?" "Yes, yes, yes! Let's go!"

"Now, lay down and close your eyes," she said. "We are in for an amazing ride, you and me!" As grandma told the story, Vincent slowly started to fall asleep. His grandma finished the story, turned off the light, and went to bed. "This was fast," she thought as Vincent dozed off.

Hours past and Vincent woke up. "What time is it?" he thought. He turned around to his nightstand to see what time it was, but his nightstand wasn't there. He looked around his room, and everything was dark. Usually, there is some light coming in from the street, but not this time. "Where is all of my furniture?!" Vincent asked. "Grandmaaaa!" he called, but here was no answer.

He got up from his bed and placed his foot onto the ground. He felt rough and hard objects under his foot. "This is not my carpet! What is this?!" Everything was dark, and he couldn't properly see where, and on what, he stood. Vincent took a step, and it made a sound as he was walking all over dried leaves. "Where am I? What is happening?" he yelled. Scared and confused, he went back to bed and covered himself over the head. "Go to sleep, go to sleep," he kept telling himself. Suddenly he heard something walking around him. "Who is out there?!" Vincent yelled. "Hh-hi...I didn't want to scare you. I've just noticed a bed in the middle of the woods, so I went over to see what it was doing out there. The bed was not alone hehe."

Vincent peeked through the covers and saw a small furry little thing circling the bed. "Hi, there!" the creature jumped on the bed as he saw Vincent peek. Vincent pulled himself to the headboard and curled. "Hi? What are you? Where am I?" he asked. "Well...first of all, my name is Perry, nice to meet you. Second of all, you are in Fairyngton – the home of all fairies," Perry explained. "Fairies? What? Fairies don't exist. Where am I?" Vincent said. "SHHHHHHHHHHH!! You can never say that again. Fairies do indeed exist, and they are the creators of everything you see here, so don't you ever repeat that again! Someone might hear you, and that won't be good." "Everything I see? But I see nothing," Vincent continued. "You will see," Perry said, "just wait until the sun comes up."

Vincent sat in complete silence while Perry continued to examine every particle of him and his bed. He was so amazed that someone different, someone human, came to his world. And Vincent – he was still so confused. Questions about how he got here were constantly roaming through his mind. He wasn't home anymore. "Someone must have taken my bed and me and left us here, in the woods, where wild mushrooms grow, so they gave me hallucinations, and that's how Perry appeared," Vincent kept on thinking about all of the different scenarios which could've to happen.

The sun has started to rise, and the rays were shining through the trees. "Oh wow, sparkles? Fruits? Colors? This is so different than it is at night. And why is everything so small?" Vincent asked. "Well, the Fairyngton was made for fairies and small creatures. Since they all are small, the things that they have or need are small, too. I am one of the biggest creatures here, and I am a lot smaller than you. So, try to imagine how others look like," Perry said. Vincent looked around to see if he could find anything to eat. "I'm so hungry," he mumbled. "Well, why don't you say so!" Perry jumped. He ran away as fast as he could and left Vincent looking, again, all confused. Minutes passed, and Vincent saw Perry running towards him with a basket filled with all kinds of foods. "So, I brought you bagels, strawberries, sandwiches, and cupcakes. I didn't know what you'd like, so I brought you everything I found," Perry said. "Fairies eat bagels and cupcakes?" Vincent asked. "Well, yes. They make them, and they eat them. They are pretty small, but you will never try better cupcakes than these, right here, trust me!"

Vincent took a bite. "Oh, WOW!!! These are amazing!!" he yelled pretty loudly. At the same moment, a flock of birds flew over them at a fast pace. "What just happened? Was I too loud?" Vincent asked. "No, no, it wasn't you. But it's better if we go someplace else. Maybe my house. I'll tell you all about it when we get there."

They walked a while and got to Perry's house. "Wait here for a bit. I have to talk to my mom about you staying with us." Vincent looked around and wasn't even sure how he would fit through the door. "OK, the coast is clear you can come in now. Just bend down a little, and you'll fit right through." Vincent managed to enter the house somehow, but there weren't any chairs big enough for him. He sat on the floor and looked at Perry and his family. They were like nothing he's seen before. Perry moved his chair closer to Vincent and started telling him why they had to leave the place where Vincent woke up.

"Not a while ago, someone ate all of our food. All of the blackberries were gone. The corn and all of the lettuce were half-eaten, now we only have strawberries and the baked goods that we've made before all the veggies were gone," Perry said. "That's horrible! Do you know who did it?" Vincent asked. "No, and we will probably never find out. The fairies led an investigation, but no one was found. And now, even though it hasn't happened again, the guard is roaming around the forest and

248

locking up everyone who is new here. Unfortunately, since we are so small, we won't be able to cover all of the fruit and vegetable fields before the winter, so we have to manage what we have now."

Vincent was so sad to hear Perry's story. Even though the citizens of Fairyngton had to limit their meals, Perry brought him a basket filled with foods in the morning. "How can I help?" asked Vincent. "I was so hungry this morning and you've brought me enough food to feed a small village. I want to repay you. My hands are a lot bigger than yours are, and I can plant seeds faster than you can. We can get the work done before winter." "Oh no, I couldn't ask you to do that. That would be too much," Perry said.

Vincent insisted on his offer, and Perry and his family eventually agreed. The next day, they went to the Fairy, who was in charge of the planting and the food Mivela. Mivela said she would accept Vincent's offer only if Perry and his family would guarantee for him. "How do we know he isn't the one who ate all of our food? He sure is big enough to do it," said Mivela. Perry explained how Vincent got to Farrington days after the eating incident happened, so there was no way he could've done it. Mivela approved, and they've agreed on the date of the planting. "The planting will start the day after tomorrow and will have to be done by the end of the week."

At the day of the planting, all of the Farrington and Vincent met at the fields and started planting the seeds. It was obvious that Vincent was faster and was able to cover more grounds than anyone else. By the evening, he was done with most of the fruits, and the next day moved on to vegetables. He finished all the work in 3 days – 2 days sooner than Mivela said. "Bravo, bravo!" cheered Farrington. "Thank you, Vincent. You've helped us so much, and now Farrington and all of his citizens are safe because of you. There will be no hunger, and everyone will have more than enough. Thank you so much!" said Mivela. The whole Farrington celebrated with a festival and made a gift for their hero. "This is for you, Vincent. The largest basket we have, with the best food we could pick out," said Farrington.

After the festival, Vincent and Perry went back to Vincent's bed. "Thank you for letting me stay at your house, but I think I'm a bit too big, and I take up too much space. I've noticed your mom can't even pass by me on her way to the kitchen," they both laughed. Perry left home, and Vincent went to bed. It was the same bed he woke up in when he got to this strange place. As he was falling asleep, he thought about how much fun he had and how many friends he made. He was never this happy and felt so proud of how he helped them.

The next morning Vincent woke up, feeling fresh and satisfied, but something was different. "Hey, am I home?!" he yelled. His grandma appeared on his doorstep. "What's the matter, Vincent? Did you have a nightmare?" she asked. He soon realized he was back in his room with all of his furniture and toys. "No, grandma. I had the best dream ever!" said Vincent. As they were heading to the kitchen for breakfast, he told her where he was and what he did. "See Vincent – remember when I told you, you were in for an amazing ride – and you were!" she smiled and continued walking towards the kitchen.

CHAPTER 17

The Golden Fairy

A long time ago, in the fairyland, golden fairies were hard to find. They were very special fairies and often carried out special tasks. Apart from their golden color, they were the only fairies able to grow the most important possession of any fairy, which was the fairy dust. They only came out on special occasions, especially at the beginning of different seasons.

The fairies were given the responsibility of growing flowers in the summer; their job was to grow several colors of flowers seen around the gardens. They could only grow these flowers with their fairy dust, but no colored fairy could get the fairy dust without the golden fairies. The coming of a golden fairy signified the beginning of summer, and this was a period the colored fairies looked forward to.

The fairies were of various colors, blue, red, purple, green and yellow. All the colored fairies were trained to tend and grow flowers, but the golden fairies were in charge of distributing the fairy dust to the various fairies at the beginning of the summer.

The golden fairy travelled long distances to distribute this fairy dust.

One day, as the golden fairy travelled to several fairy villages to distribute the fairy dust at the start of the summer, she came about an old carriage. The carriage was ridden by an old man in an oversized jacket. The carriage was also being driven by two black horses. The golden fairy went up to the horses and smoothened their mane. Her hands felt cold on the horses' nose. It was a very beautiful horse.

"Wheeeey. " The horse shouted at the sight of the golden fairy. The horse had never seen a fairy before.

"What is wrong with you boy?! Keep still!" The coachman said to his horse. The horse kept galloping all around the hilly road, almost throwing the driver from its back. The horse was riding wildly because he was disturbed by the sight of the golden fairy. The golden fairy wished she didn't have to continue flying and sharing the fairy dust from one fairy village to another. It was not an easy job. She had to fly to faraway places.

"I wish I didn't have to fly about sharing the fairy dust every summer. I would love to sit around doing nothing but looking at the sun and flying around like the colored fairies." The golden fairy said. She was tired of flying with the big load of fairy dust carried at her back. Then the golden fairy decided to ride in the carriage secretly. She gently placed her bag of fairy dust in the corner of the carriage. Using it as a pillow, the golden fairy slept off to the gentle sway of the moving carriage. The next morning, the golden fairy knew that there was something different about her environment. This was not the same place she had slept the previous night. There was no window and no horse. She looked around but could see nothing.

"Where am I?" she wondered. She searched around for the sac of fairy dust she had placed underneath herself when she was about to sleep. It was not there anymore, and this worried her. Without the sac of golden dust, there would be no summer flowers.

"What would I do? the fairy dust is gone!" The golden fairy cried. She tried her best to get out of the room she was, but there was no means of exit. The golden fairy began hitting the walls of the room.

"Let me out! Let me out!" She shouted. Suddenly, a small window was opened. The golden fairy could see someone peeping through the small hole.

"Who are you, and what have you done with my fairy dust?" She asked angrily. There was a wild laugh coming from the other end of the box. The golden fairy listened closely to what they were saying. She had never heard them before.

"I would never have thought that fairies were real until I saw one," a loud voice said. "She is indeed, very beautiful. I wonder where she came from. I am so lucky that I found this rare creature in my carriage."

"I can't wait until everyone sees her. They will pay lots of money just to see her. We would be rich." Another person said. The golden fairy listened carefully to their statements. It seemed she had been captured by the humans and kept in a box.

"Oh my!" she cried. She had slept in the carriage because she was tired. She never planned on being seen by humans. The fairies were usually very careful not to be seen by anyone. But now, she had been caught and would be shown to other humans for money. The other fairies would surely be unhappy with her. "Who would share the fairy dust this summer? And how would the flowers grow?" The golden fairy worried.

"Let me out now! Let me out! " The golden fairy shouted as loud as her voice could go. The golden fairy stayed in that little box for several weeks, and these weeks became months. The box was not comfortable for a fairy. Fairies were meant to fly and not to sit in a box. Every day she felt sad and wished she could be back with the other fairies doing her job of sharing the fairy dust. She wished she had not slept in that carriage.

The golden fairy was taken to a big human carnival filled with so many humans with painted faces, singing and dancing. The golden fairy was placed in a glass box.

"Leave me alone." She shouted when one of the humans tried picking her up. Of course, the humans did not understand what she was saying because they did not understand fairy language. While one of the humans tried to touch her, she bit him hard on his fingers.

253

"Ouch!" He shouted. When she was eventually placed in the glass box, her golden light filled the whole place like a lamp. The humans in the carnival paid lots of money to touch her.

"Go away!" she would shout. The humans would clap and cheer at her sight. They loved seeing the beautiful golden light that shone brightly from her.

Later at night, the old man in the oversized jacket would ask her to go to sleep and cover up her glass box with a thick blanket. She felt sad and lonely because she really missed the other fairies and her job. She thought about what they would be doing in fairyland when they notice her absence. She hoped that they would search for her.

The old man in the oversized jacket kept taking her from one carnival to another and she feared that soon she would travel too far away from the fairyland. Then there would be no summer plants growing. The golden fairy tried to sleep when suddenly, her glass box began to shake violently. The golden fairy pressed her ears to the glass, trying to hear what was happening.

"Take it with the blanket." She heard a man's voice say. Some men were stealing her. They were taking her away from the old man with an oversized jacket. The men took her on their horse and rode away. They rode so fast that the golden fairy felt horse sick. They rode far into the night and far away from the carnival. The golden fairy did not like these men. They placed her under the hot sun during the day, and at night she would be placed in a large room with so many men studying her and trying to understand her. They had never seen a fairy before.

"She is speaking some kind of fairy language. No one can understand her," One of the men said. She was being examined with a big magnifying glass.

"I wonder what makes her glow." Another said. The golden fairy listened to them talk. She had to find a way to get away from them.

Back in fairyland, the fairies were very worried. The golden fairy was supposed to have come around and shared the fairy dust, but no one had heard from her.

"Summer is here already, and the golden fairy is yet to arrive." A red fairy said. The fairies had called for a meeting of all the fairies to discuss the absence of the golden fairy. There were no plants around and soon; humans would begin to wonder why the plants were not growing.

"The golden fairy is too proud." Another fairy said. "It is sad that at this time she is yet to share the fairy dust to us. I think that we could ask fairies in all the fairy villages so as to know exactly if the golden fairy had given them any fairy dust to grow flowers this summer." the fairies sent word around and it was discovered that the golden fairy had not visited any of the fairy villages.

"There will be no flowers of any color at all this summer." a yellow fairy said sadly. Soon the fairies heard about the carnivals where the golden fairy had been. The golden fairy had become very popular among humans.

"It's said that the golden fairy left us so she can attend the carnival. She has forgotten that it is not allowed for a fairy to be seen by a human." the fairies cried. They did not know that the golden fairy had been captured by the humans, instead, they thought that the golden fairy had chosen to leave them. The fairies decided to send some of their brave and strong fairies to go and meet with the golden fairy. The fairies all had strong wings that could fly long distances. The poor golden fairy was so tired of staying in the glass box.

One day, a big dog strolled into the place where the golden fairy was kept. He loved the light shining from the glass box. The golden fairy started hitting the glass box until the dog got so interested in the glowing glass and knocked it off the shelf. The box fell to the ground and shattered. The dog tried to pick up the glowing fairy to his mouth, but the golden fairy quickly flew off very far into the air. She flew very high, circling the place severally because she was happy to be free again.

"Yuhooo! I am free." The golden fairy shouted. She was happy until she remembered that they had taken the fairy dust. "There is no fairy dust, so there would be no flowers this summer. " the golden fairy said to herself. She began flying back as fast as she could to the fairyland. She knew that by now, the other fairies would be very worried. As the golden fairy was flying again, the brave fairies sent from the fairyland searched everywhere for the fairy. They saw the broken glass box on the ground, but there was no golden fairy.

"The golden fairy is gone." One of the fairies said sadly.

"We would never get our fairy dust to grow our flowers again." Another fairy said. The brave fairies sadly flew back home. At that time, the golden fairy had arrived in the fairyland.

"Where have you been? There is no fairy dust to grow our flowers. We all know that you went to the carnival." They said. The golden fairy told them the story of how she was captured by the old man in the oversized jacket and then stolen from him by other humans. The fairies listened quietly to the golden fairy's story.

"What are we going to do about the fairy dust? If we don't get more fairy dust, our fields would not have flowers." After hearing this, the golden fairy had an idea. She decided to make another.

"It took a whole year to make the last fairy dust; you would never be able to make it all in time for the summer." A fairy said.

"We would if we work as a team." The golden fairy said. She divided the fairies into groups. Some fairies had the task of fetching the materials that would be used to make the fairy dust. The second group were to perform the ritual dance to make the dust. Others build fairy sacs for the dust. All the fairies had something important to do. They watched the golden fairy dance so hard. She would dance and fly, dance and fly,

256

making beautiful patterns in the air. Gradually the fairy dust began to form. They worked really hard, day and night until they completed the fairy dust. The fairies were very happy. They had made something beautiful through teamwork and hard work. All the fairies were given a portion of the fairy dust to grow their flowers.

They grew their flowers as quickly as they could. From that day, the golden fairy promised always to make the fairy dust available on time. They worked as a team year after year, and they lived happily ever after.

THE END

CHAPTER 18

Dynamo The Dragon

The sun was high in the sky as Alex and Tanum climbed the forested mountain. They were not only best friends; they were also explorers. Together, they had discovered much of the world together. Everywhere they went, they brought backpacks full of books, papers, and pencils to record their findings. Whenever they set out for a new adventure, they never knew what they were going to find.

But today was different.

After a few hours of hiking, Alex and Tanum decided to take a break at a large boulder. A break in the clouds above allowed big glowing beams of sunlight to fall upon their village in the valley far below. While Alex looked out over the edge, Tanum set down his backpack and removed an old book from the inside.

"Says here this area used to be full of dragon caves," said Tanum. "If Dynamo exists, he probably lives around here."

Alex laughed.

"Don't be silly, Tanum," he replied. "Dynamo does not exist. Dragons do not exist. You should know that. There has not been a single dragon seen in over a hundred thousand years. Just enjoy the adventure!"

With that, Alex took out a dark leather-bound notebook and began to sketch a drawing of the valley far below. He drew the stormy clouds and the sunlight that fell through them. He drew the tall, dark pines and the ring of mountains in the distance and the river that flowed from their rocky peaks to pass by their village.

While Alex drew, Tanum looked around. He was not so sure that Alex was right. Over the last few days, there had been numerous stories of strange sounds echoing out from the mountains. One of the villagers even claimed to have seen something huge flying through the sky late one night.

"C'mon," Tanum told Alex. "I think it would be best if we kept moving."

They put away their things and continued their hike up the mountain. As they climbed, Tanum kept his eyes out, and his ears open. But all he could hear were birds twittering in the trees and critters scurrying in the undergrowth. Once, they saw a fox chasing a possum into a burrow, but other than that, there was nothing out of the ordinary.

Then, suddenly, Alex raised a hand.

"Shhh," he hissed. "Do you hear that?"

They had just come around a bend into a large, sunlit clearing. Tanum leaned against his walking stick and listened, but all that he could hear was the chirping of the birds in the trees.

"I do not hear anything," said Tanum.

"Listen closer."

Again, Tanum turned his attention to the outside world. Then he heard it. Above the sound of birds and the wind blowing through the trees, there came a slow, deep rumble. The sound was faint, but it seemed to cause the stones and the trunks of the trees around them to tremble.

Alex looked scared.

"I have never heard anything like it," he said. "What do you think it is?"

"I don't know," said Tanum. "But it's coming from up there."

Tanum pointed to the slope beside them; it was covered in the shade of towering pine trees. At the very top was a rocky ridge.

259

"Should we investigate?" Alex asked.

"Absolutely."

The hill was very steep. There was no trail for them to follow, so they had to climb slowly and carefully. Even so, the way was not easy. Twice, Alex stepped on loose rocks and almost tumbled down the slope, and Tanum brushed a bush of poison ivy that left his legs itching and scratching. When they reached the middle of the hill, Alex stopped and suggested that they forget the whole thing and return to the path where it was safe. But Tanum waved his idea away. He was so interested in the sound coming from the ridge above them that he could think of nothing else.

Was this the sound that the villagers had talked about? Did it belong to the massive winged creature spotted in the night? Was it Dynamo?

When they reached the top of the slope, they found two bears sleeping in the sun beneath the rocky ridge.

"There you go," said Alex. "Two bears, no dragons. Are you happy Tanum?"

Tanum tried hushing his friend, but it was too late. The bears had heard him. Grumbling, they raised their heads, sniffing at the air. When they saw Alex and Tanum standing close to their den, they growled and rose to their feet.

"Run!" Tanum yelled.

It was too risky to run back down the slope, so instead, they ran around the ridge, jumping over stones and climbing over the boulders. When they were sure they had escaped, they stopped.

"Where are we?" Asked Alex, panting.

They had reached a long stony plateau.

"I don't know."

260

"Great," said Alex, dropping his backpack on the ground. "I hope you are happy, Tanum. Because of your dragon seeking, we may have gotten ourselves lost!"

This made Tanum angry.

"Don't blame me. You are the one who woke the bears up!"

Alex opened his pack and started looking for a map.

"Don't even try to blame this on me. If you had not forced us up that stupid hill looking for a dragon, we would not have had to run in the first place!"

Tanum grew red in the face.

"I was not looking for a dragon."

"Yes, you were, Tanum," said Alex running out of patience. "How many times do I have to tell you. It is so simple. Dragons do not—"

"Shhh," Tanum hissed. "Do you hear that?"

Alex scrunched his face together, listening. After a moment, a look of disbelief crossed his eyes.

"Yes," he said slowly. "It's that sound again."

Over the sound of their footsteps and breathing, they had not been able to hear it, but the sound was still there.

"It wasn't the bears," said Tanum. "It was something else."

Alex looked around.

"Where is it coming from?"

Tanum pointed

"Right there."

Hidden in the shade of numerous pines, right in the middle of a tall rock face, yawned an enormous cave.

"Didn't you say dragons lived in caves?" said Alex.

"Yes," said Tanum. "Yes, I did. C'mon, let's check it out."

"We just got chased by bears, and now, you want to get chased by a dragon?!"

But it was too late. Tanum was already running toward the cave. He paused just outside the mouth, waiting for Alex to catch up. Somewhere within the darkness came the slow, deep rumbling.

"Let us light a torch," said Alex. "Or we won't be able to see anything."

When their torches were lit, they ventured forward into the cave. Inside, they stood and looked around. Firelight danced off the glistening cave walls, and somewhere in the distance came the drip drip drip of water.

Alex pointed toward another opening on the far side of the cave.

"The sound is coming from over there," he whispered.

Very quietly and very carefully, Alex and Tanum made their way toward the other opening. Beyond was a massive tunnel descending into darkness.

Tanum looked at Alex.

"Just a quick peek, and we'll be out of here."

Alex nodded.

Torches clasped firmly in hand, they made their way down the tunnel. They were very careful not to make any noise. The smallest stone sounded like a thunderstorm in here. With each step they took, the rumbling below grew louder in their ears. But now, it was mixed with something else—the sharp clink of metal against stone. The tunnel began to grow warm around them. Tanum placed his hand against the stone and was not surprised to feel small tremors.

"We are getting closer."

Finally, the tunnel opened into a spacious cavern. When Tanum and Alex stepped forward, they could hardly believe their eyes. The fire from their torches glinted off enormous mounds of golden coins, heaps of precious gemstones, and racks of jewel-encrusted armor and artifacts. Curled up on top of all of it was a massive, sleeping dragon. Even his scales looked like precious metals, and with each new breath, he sent objects scattering about the cave.

"Is that Dynamo?" Alex whispered, eyes the size of dinner plates.

Tanum dropped to one knee and pulled out his dragon book. He brushed through the pages.

"Yes," he said, glancing between the dragon and a page in the book. "That is—that is Dynamo!"

"Incredible."

Tanum closed the book and carefully put it away. At the same moment, Dynamo decided to stretch his leg, sending a spray of golden coins and other objects in their direction. For a moment, before he nestled his head back into a pile of treasure, Tanum caught a glimpse of eyes like red-hot embers.

"Incredible. Definitely." Tanum rose shakily to his feet. "Anyway, we have seen our dragon. I think it would be best if we let him sleep."

"Hold on, hold on," Alex whispered. "Let us hang back and draw a picture!"

"No," Tanum hissed. "No, I do not think that would be a good idea."

Dynamo rumbled, and the cave filled with blistering heat.

"Fine," said Alex, sweat dotting his forehead. "But let us take something then—a souvenir so that we can remember our adventure."

"I said just one quick peek. We have already done that; now, let us get out of here before something bad happens!"

Tanum turned from his friend and began climbing back up the tunnel. When Tanum looked back, Alex was not there. He was about to turn back for his friend when he appeared a moment later, adjusting his backpack.

"Hold on, wait for me!"

When they stepped out of the cave a few minutes later, the sun was already sinking toward the horizon. By the time they found the trail again, dark shadows were growing between the trees.

"I guess you were right about dragons," said Alex. "I am sorry that I did not believe you."

Every second step, Tanum heard something clink inside of Alex's backpack. But that could have been anything.

"Do not worry about it," said Tanum. "I'm sorry I yelled at you. If you had not woken the bears, we would never have found the dragon!"

With that, they continued their journey down the trail. Every time they came around a bend in the trail, they were able to glimpse the shingled roofs of their village through the trees, and each time again, the village looked a little closer. Soon, they would be home, and Tanum would write about everything he had seen.

They were about halfway down when suddenly, a great roar halted them in their tracks. The sound echoed over the mountains and across the valley, shaking them to the bone. The sound was deep and sorrowful and sad.

"What was that?" Alex asked, looking scared.

264

"I don't know," replied Tanum. "Maybe a bear?"

That seemed to cheer up his friend, and together they went on walking, laughing, and joking, tall pines creaking in the wind around them.

Through the trees, the village walls loomed up out of the undergrowth. The guards at the gate recognized them and let them pass with a solemn nod of their heads.

"Welcome back, youngins," grunted one of the guards.

"Discover anything new out there today?" Asked the other.

"Not much," said Tanum. "Just a dragon's cave."

The guards laughed.

"Dragon, ye say?" said the first.

"Shoulda brought me home some scales!" said the second. "My wife's been bugging me for a new dress all year!"

While the guards roared with laughter, Tanum and Alex entered the village, grinning. They knew that nobody would believe them. But that did not matter because they could find the cave anytime they wanted.

"I'm going back to my place," said Tanum. "I've got a lot of writing to do."

"Me too," said Alex. "A lot of drawings."

With that, the two friends parted ways, each back to his own house.

Tanum discovered his house dark and empty. A scribbled note on the kitchen table read that his mother would be at his aunt's house until later that evening. Tanum folded the letter, tucked it away into a drawer, and went to his room to find his curtains drawn over the window. To spook the chill darkness, he threw them open and lit several tallow candles. Then, sitting most comfortably at his desk, Tanum withdrew his notebook and quills from his bag and set them down in front of him.

From a drawer, Tanum removed a pair of wiry spectacles and fixed them upon his eyes. Flexing his fingers, he inked his quill and set it down upon a fresh piece of parchment.

The quill began to scribble.

Tanum wrote everything that he was able to remember: the hike up the trail and the various creatures they encountered along the way, including the owl that nearly got stuck in his hair at the beginning of the hike. He wrote about their climb up the hill, the slips and the stumbles, the poison ivy, and the two bears, which led them to Dynamo the Dragon's cave.

Tanum was setting down the quill to begin the next sentence, when a roar, much like the one they had heard on their way down from the mountain, made him stop.

That's odd, Tanum thought to himself.

When the echo faded and the soft trill of crickets and murmuring voices in the market swelled to take its place, Tanum lowered his quill to the parchment and began scribbling again.

After lighting their torches, Tanum and Alex had entered the cave and descended the dark tunnel into Dynamo's lair. Tanum remembered the great heaps of glinting treasure and the enormous dragon that lay sprawled over the top. Dynamo's scales had shone in the torchlight, and in the gloom, his eyes had looked like burning coals. At that moment, as he stood there, staring into Dynamo's eyes, Tanum had felt smaller than an ant. Promising that he would never do anything to get on Dynamo's bad side, Tanum turned to leave the cave. Alex had lagged behind—

Another roar echoed down from the mountain, this time closer. Something about the roar made Tanum set down his quill and rush to his backpack. From within, he withdrew his dragon book and flipped through its pages.

"Here it is…" he mumbled.

266

CHAPTER 19

The Princess Under the Sea

There once was a lovely young woman who lived in the sea. She was born in the sea and knew only of its properties and its abundance. Her father was the King of the Realm, and guarded her aggressively, as he loved her more than life itself.

Her name was Ari, and she was a mermaid. Ari often swam close to the land and then popped up to the surface to watch the men on the beach and in the neighboring town. She was lonely and had begun to feel restless with her life under the sea. She wanted so very badly to walk like the land women she saw on the beach and to find a landman who would love her and want to take care of her forevermore.

One day, she went to see her Fathers Sorcerer and told him about her dreams and her desires. The Sorcerer was aware that the King had bid her never to even speak of the land species, and that to ever leave the safety of the water was never going to be allowed. He knew that, and she knew that, but nevertheless, he came up with a plan, and on the following week, he called Ari to his chamber.

Ari was intrigued by the Sorcerers plan and became very excited. She had been spending more time watching the people on the beach than ever, and she knew that she would never be happy until she was able to go forth unto the world of the walking and find her mate. She listened carefully, as the wicked Sorcerer outlined his plan and agreed to all of its terms. The plan was kept a secret from the King, as she knew her Father would lock her in her chamber for an eternity if he found out. She had the Sorcerer make up a potion that she would drink and would become a landlady, but there was a catch. She would only be able to stay a landlady for a period of one week before she would again turn into a mermaid.

On the day she had set aside to swim to the water's edge and then drink the potion, she made herself look as pretty as she possibly could, and then left the King's domain. As she swam nearer to the water's edge, she became nervous. "What if the potion does not work, and I get stuck on the land forever? What if the potion does not work, and I become old and ugly and stuck on the land forever?" she thought. Then she said to herself, "You are just being silly. The King's Sorcerer is the finest Sorcerer, and he would never make such a ridiculous mistake."

Ari swam on her back for some time going over what it would be like to be human, and to walk on two legs, and do human things like fall in love. "Fall in love," she whispered to herself; "Fall in love?" yes, that is what she wanted, so she would go ahead and drink the potion. With that, she pulled out the vial the Sorcerer had given her and drank the entire thing down. Then, she began to feel very strange but in a very good way. Her vision blurred for the moment, and she felt light-headed and drifty. Then, everything changed, and she felt as though she had been sleeping for all of her life and not had woken up. She felt elated, alive, and excited all at the same time.

Ari looked around at the beach again; only this time, the beach looked like where she would have to go if she wanted to go home, and the deep ocean looked like a place to go if she wanted to explore. "The potion has worked beyond all my expectations!" she thought to herself. "And now, for the ultimate test of its power," she thought as she looked down at her tail. The tail was nowhere to be seen and in its place were two long, slender, and beautiful legs. "This will do nicely!" she exclaimed aloud, "Very nicely."

She immediately began swimming for the shore, and for the very first time in all of her years, she put her feet down and felt the sandy bottom, the sand between her toes, and the movement of legs and feet. Something she had been dreaming about for so very long. Then another

268

first. Ari was now in the shallow waters near the very edge of the ocean, where it meets the sandy beach. She looked at the beach now only a matter of feet from her and watched as the water lapped up and down on the seashore. It was a beautiful sight to her as she could never have come this close to land before when she had a tail instead of these two wonderful legs, as she could have easily become stranded and then discovered by the humans. Everyone had warned all the children in the realm that if the humans ever caught them, they would poke and prod them and put them in cages and treat them like a freak. "Nobody should ever have to endure such treatment," the king had taught them.

But now, she could easily just walk out of the water and up the beach and talk to whomever she pleased. Her time had come, and so, for the very first time in her life, she placed her two new feet on the sandy bottom, leaned forward to put all of her body weight over them and pushed up. She was standing. For the very first time in her life, she was actually standing, and she loved this new feeling. "This is great!" she called out aloud. "What is great?" a man's voice nearby asked. Ari was shocked and stunned. She had never ever heard a real man's voice spoken over the air of the planet. She turned to see an old man wearing a pair of ugly bathing trunks standing not 20 feet from her. "Oh, hello," she said. "I was just planning a party for my husband," she lied, "And I thought of a great way to surprise him." She continued. "Oh, so it's a surprise party, eh?" the man muttered. "What? Oh Uh... yes, that's right. A surprise party for my husband." And then she turned and walked for the very first time. She walked like a real woman that she indeed was on that day. She walked with confidence. She walked with character and charisma.

"But where was she walking to?" she began to wonder. "Oh no," she thought. "I did not think this through very well. Now, what do I do?" she asked herself.

She saw a small building with a palm leaf roof and noticed that there were a lot of people sitting on high chairs and leaning on a long platform. They were all facing the same way and laughing and talking, and most were men. "Right." She said to herself. "I'll go there and join them."

As she approached the shack, most of the men suddenly became all in a bother and began shuffling around to look at her. One of them let out a strange whistling sound that came from his mouth. "Well, hello there, sweetheart!" the closest one said. "Hey, there, honey. There's an open seat here by me. And it's open forever for you, baby!" another one claimed. She noticed all of the men were asking for her company with the exception of one. As it happened, he was way down at the other end of the platform and was very handsome. She headed towards him and was in luck. There was an open seat on the very end of the platform on the other side of the man. She walked right up to it across the sandy beach and climbed up into that high chair.

There was another man whom she had not noticed on the other side of the platform, and he had on a funny outfit. It was not a bathing suit like all the men on her side had, on but had bright red and white colors on it and was quite ugly. She tensed when she saw the strange man behind the platform walking straight towards her. "What'll it be, miss?" the man asked her. She froze. She had no idea what he was asking her or why he was even talking to her.

She just stared at him for a moment and then said, "I don't know," which was the truth. He thought she meant she didn't know what she wanted and said, "Okay, miss, I'll check back with you in a few minutes." And went back to fiddling with his glasses and bottles. The gentleman whom she had sat beside turned to look at her, and she found herself hypnotized by his bright blue eyes, his dark curly hair, and his smile.

Then he spoke. "I'm John Blake," he said, and then he waited. She knew she was supposed to say something, but she didn't know what. Her name! That was it; he wanted to meet her. Of course! "I'm Ari," she said finally and then turned to face forward again. He did not stop looking at her, and in fact, he held out his hand in a way she had never seen. His

270

thumb was facing up, and his little finger down, and his hand was stiff like a knife. She turned and made her hand into the same gesture. He looked down at both of them, holding their hands out in a ridiculous fashion and quickly took her hand with his and bobbed their hands up and down a few times and then let go of it. "How strange," she thought.

A little more time passed, and then the handsome Mr. Blake turned towards her again and said, "I was wondering if you would like to join me for a walk on the beach?" Ari's face lit up because this was something she did understand, and she liked this man very much. "I would love to," she answered with a smile. The two slid off their barstools and walked down towards the water and then down the beach. They walked and talked for over an hour and became good friends. Then, she noticed that he was a little bit nervous, and she guessed that she was too. This was wonderful. She had walked out of the water and into the life of a tall, handsome stranger.

Then suddenly, out of the blue, John asked her, "May I buy you dinner tonight?" Before she knew what, she was doing, she agreed, but there was a problem. The Sorcerer had forgotten to provide her with the whole story. She needed clothes and money and who knew what else to function on the dry land world. Realizing that she was in a bit of a jam, she quickly made up a story about how she had been on vacation with some girlfriends and had become separated from them.

That day, they were scheduled to board a bus somewhere and get to the airport, and now all she had were the clothes on her back and nowhere to stay. He bought the story and took care of everything. They went to the clothing store and purchased some fine items for her and then went to dinner. After dinner, she went home with him, and he let her stay on his couch, but before long, they fell in love, and he wanted her to stay forever. Of course, she couldn't do that but continued to make up stories about why.

Eventually, they became very happy together, and he began asking questions she had no answers for. This made her very uncomfortable,

271

so she decided to tell him the truth. "You're a Mermaid?" he said with an astonished look on his face. Ari was amazed at how well he took this incredible information and was then even more in love with him. How would they do it? What could they do to make it work now that he knew her complete truth? Then John had an idea. He told her that he was a scuba diver, and he asked her what she thought of him coming out into the water for some visits, and then she comes up on land like she was then on other visits.

That plan seemed like the only one that could possibly work. "I'll buy a sailboat," he said. "And I can pick you up, and you can be yourself and be with me on the boat. We can sail around and have lunch, and well, what do you think?" he asked. She was overjoyed at the thought of having truth between them and agreed.

In the months that followed, John and Ari spend every spare moment together. Sometimes swimming together and playing in the ocean and sometimes sailing which as it happened, she loved. She had never been on a real sailboat, and John was a great sailor. Then, one day, she went to the Sorcerer and asked him if he could change her permanently into a land walker. He was very worried about what the king would think but then figured out a way to make it, so she had control over her body. She could be herself in the water and share precious moments with her father, and she could be the land girl and be with her man whenever she liked.

Soon, John asked her to marry him, and after learning what marriage meant, she was very happy to marry him. As time went on, Ari spent most of her time with John, but just enough time with her father, so he did not suspect anything or get angry because she was spending so much time away. That was how our story went, and anyone who read it was charmed by the little girl who grew up as a Mermaid and one day actually did meet her prince charming.

In the end, she had three wonderful children, and to her relief, they all had human legs and were perfect babies. She was sad that she could not

272

tell her Father but happy that she had achieved her dreams beyond what she had ever thought possible.

Never ever let go of your dreams!

The End

CHAPTER 20

Journey With The Unicorn

B egin by lying comfortably in your bed. Take a moment to adjust your body so you feel perfectly comfortable for falling asleep. When you're ready, gently close your eyes.

You find yourself in a wide open field, on a sunny afternoon.

The lush green grass beneath your bare feet feels soft and soothing. You can feel each blade of grass tickling your toes as you walk. You bend down to lie in the grass and breathe in the refreshing fragrance of the rich, Earthy ground.

Let your body relax in this moment. Feeling the sunlight washing over you. There is not a cloud in the sky. Just a wide open expanse of sky blue air above you and the bright green grass below you.

In this moment you feel your body getting calmer and more peaceful as you hear the sound of birds singing in the distance. As their songs get louder you notice they're flying towards you. You see three silhouettes of small birds flying overhead. Their bodies are a vivid blue and their songs are mesmerizing.

You wish they'd come to visit you and as if they can hear your thoughts, they turn around in the sky and come soaring down to the ground to meet you.

You put out your hand and one at a time each little bird climbs into your hand, and up your arm. Once all three are on your arm, you feel called to stand up and walk with them. Their songs continue to lull you into a feeling of peace and serenity. They feel so loving and kind, like they really care about you.

You feel so happy having these new bird friends with you, you ask them which way they'd like to go. With that question two of them fly ahead of you while one stays on your shoulder. You know they are leading the way and you begin to follow them.

As you walk through the grassy field, following these two beautiful bright blue birds, you look down and notice a snail on a tall blade of grass. His shell is a vivid red and yellow swirl.

It feels like there is so much magic in this field. Even though you aren't exactly sure why, you feel like these birds are leading you to something truly wondrous.

You begin to get closer to the edge where the field meets a large green forest with thick, wide and ancient-looking trees. Every tree in this forest looks wide enough to be able to be hollowed out and turned into a home for you, or perhaps for fairies. You start to wonder, maybe that's exactly what they are!

The birds lead you to a trail at the beginning of the forest. The path is lined with silver glittering sparkles. Even though the path is well shaded from the sun because of the massive, giant trees, the path still glimmers as if the sun was beaming down on it. The path is so bright and illustrious you have to squint your eyes at first.

It feels like all the trees around you are welcoming you into their forest.

So as you take your first step on the sparkling glittering trail, you feel a wave of deep peace and comfort wash over you.

Take a moment to notice how your body relaxes into this.

You begin to walk along the trail, all three of the birds now flying in front of you.

You notice that the birds fly up into a tree up ahead. Curious, you follow them to the tree, placing your hands the rough and peeling pale brownish grey bark. This tree is so wide it takes you several steps to walk all the way around it. You can tell there is something glowing behind this tree.

Your eagerness and excitement to discover what is glowing guides your way as you finally make your way around the tree until you are face to face with the magic you knew you felt in this place.

There are you, standing right in front of a pure white and shimmering unicorn. Her horn is a radiant pearlescent spiral and her mane and tail glisten just like the silvery sparkles in the path that led you to her.

She emanates a calming, and soothing presence.

You feel so relaxed and comfortable standing before her - as if you've known her all your life, and the two are you are dear old friends.

She bows down her head and you slowly walk over and gently place your hand on her nose.

You can feel the warmth of her breath as you lean in your head to rest on hers.

The two of you take a few deep and relaxing breaths together. Feeling the peacefulness that being together brings.

As your breathing slows, softens and deepens, she kneels down all the way so that you can climb onto her back.

Her hair feels silky smooth and warm to the touch, as if she's been bathing in the sun. You find it easy to climb up on her, getting one leg on either side and wrapping your arms around her neck. As you do this, you bury your head deep into her mane and take a long inhale. She smells almost like freshly baked cookies or cake. You can't quite put your finger on it, but it's a comforting and welcome scent.

276

Once you are safely holding on to her, she stands up and begins to walk very slowly. She trots at a very gentle pace to help you get acquainted and comfortable holding on to her back. You find the gentle rocking back and forth of holding on to her to be soothing and peaceful.

She can sense that you are getting more comfortable and so she starts to gallop at a faster speed. The wind comes flowing over your face and you're surprised at how smooth this feels. So you look down and notice - she's lifted off the ground. She's flying!

There's an opening between the trees up ahead where you can see the bright, clear sky and you can tell that she's headed directly towards that opening.

You can hear the leaves in the trees rustling as you get closer to the skyline.

As you look down you can see the little birds waving their wings as if to say good-bye for now.

And with that the two of you fly through the treeline and enter into the wide, open sky.

It feels like freedom as the wind blows all over your skin and your clothes. The Unicorn's mane is whipping in the wind all around you - causing you to see almost nothing but bright silvery sparkles.

Because of her mane and the distraction of the sparkles, you can't tell exactly where you're headed.

But you can feel the freedom of the sky, and comfort of flying.

And suddenly you notice more than just the sparkles all around you from your Unicorn's mane - now you see bright, white, fluffy clouds.

You think to yourself, "where did these come from? The sky was so clear before?"

It's as if you've been transported into a cloud world - for all around you are fluffy white clouds, and Unicorns walking around on them. There are benches made of rainbows where you see friends and family sitting and relaxing in this magical space.

You feel so safe and loved here.

Your Unicorn kneels down to help you hop off.

And as you step onto the soft, fluffy clouds, your feet feel as if they are hardly touching anything. It feels like you are floating.

You walk this way, with your hand on your Unicorns front leg - the two of you walking through this cloud land together.

It feels like every single step you take brings you more peace and comfort.

You start to feel very tired and relaxed, so your Unicorn leads you to one of the rainbow benches for you to lie down on.

You walk past blue unicorns, and red unicorns and unicorns of every color - all with their manes and tails glistening in the sunlight.

As you reach an open bench made out of a radiant rainbow, you're surprised to find that it is warm and cozy to the touch. It almost feels like a soft, fluffy blanket. As you sit down you notice your body feels so soothed and protected. You lift up your legs and lie down comfortably on the bench. It feels like this bench has a magical ability to make you feel more comfortable than you've ever felt before.

Your Unicorn bows her head to nuzzle your face, as if to wish you good night.

The rainbow bench wraps you up in rainbow light, as if a warm blanket is tucking you in. You feel so peaceful, safe and loved here.

There is a deeply soothing and relaxing energy in this space and you notice your breathing as slowed, your body as relaxed and your mind feels ready for dreams.

As you relax more and more, you start to feel yourself drifting off into the deepest, more peaceful sleep. Your Unicorn gives you the gift of having beautiful dreams while you sleep tonight. And you let yourself drift off into a perfect night of rest.

CHAPTER 21

Mouse of Doom

The animal keepers at The Funmazing Circus thought that they were so clever when they named the new baby elephant Eleanor. However, Eleanor the Elephant is a mouthful and they have regretted it evermore.

Eleanor (Ellen for short) was the most adorable baby animal that the performers had ever seen. She was the color of clouds before a storm and tripped over her own ears more than anyone has ever tripped over anything. She was a bubbly little creature and would never shy away from learning new tricks. Ellen wore a periwinkle bow around her neck because she had always loved the color. A few of the trainers lamented that she was the sassiest little elephant and deserved her own hour in the show to perform her tricks. Ellen loved her job in the circus and had a natural presence on the stage. She was also a huge draw for the crowds, and they used her image on all the printed advertisements. Ellen had learned a new trick where she would lay down behind a large board that served as a wall to block her body. One of the trainers would play snake-charming music, and she would allow her trunk to slowly dance up above the wooden wall. The audience would think that she was a snake. She and the trainer would keep this illusion going for quite a while before she would stand up and reveal herself to the audience. They would scream and applaud her so loudly. She would stumble off the main stage, accidentally stepping on her ears once or three times.

Ellen was a wonderful performer and loved her life with her circus family. One fateful day, the trainers told her that she needed to work on her grace and balance. She was understandably upset. Ellen was a star!

The audience seemed to love her exactly as she was, so why were they asking her to do something that was in opposition to her nature? It wasn't like they were asking her to do a new trick, they were asking her to change her nature. This brought Ellen to the point of tears and she felt as though they were telling her that she wasn't good enough. She didn't take the revelation well and ran to her specialized enclosure to sulk. The peppy pink and purple colors that adorned her walls were not enough to lift her spirits at this moment, as they had been in the past. She buried her head in a pillow and enclosed her ears around her, in a further effort to drown out the world around her.

Ellen sobbed for a while, knowing that's important to allow oneself to express one's emotions. As she began to calm down, she noticed a rustling in the stillness of her room. A tiny noise penetrated the quiet and caused the small elephant to take pause. She slowly pulled her ears from over her eyes to find the culprit. The movement stopped and Ellen decided that it must have just been the wind playing tricks on her very sensitive hearing. All the tears had worn our young hero completely out, so she repositioned her ears and readied herself for a nap. No sooner than she had covered her eyes again, that darn noise came back. She was determined to find the source, so she moved slowly and methodically this time. Ellen allowed her ears to gently fall away from her face, as though she were asleep. The tiny disturbance paused for a moment and then continued, probably safe in the knowledge that the elephant was resting. That is when she saw the creature responsible for the ruckus and her heart sank. It is at this point in our story that we must take a moment to understand a crucial fact about elephants. They have a natural aversion to small animals. This is a widely accepted fact, but we must understand why. In the chaos of excitement, it would be very easy for a tiny creature to misplace its' sense of direction and run right up an elephant's trunk. It is speculated that elephants are born with this disdain for smallness, and object to a tiny thing in the same way that you or I might object to a snake or a spider.

A small brown mouse stood anxiously in the corner of the room, looking for leftover straw for her own house. This tiny mouse had a nerve of steel and was mostly unbothered by the elephant while trying to be very mindful of its' awareness. She was a scavenger of other's junk but was also very careful not to take anything of sentimental value to anyone else. The tiny mouse occasionally glanced up at Ellen, and finally realized that she was being watched. They both let out a terrible shriek and the mouse scurried away in a blind panic. Ellen was still frozen with fear and concerned that the mouse might return to finish what it started. She stayed glued to her pillow for some time before she gathered her courage and went to find her trainer. The trainers searched her room from top to bottom and found no evidence that a mouse was ever there. They assumed that the small elephant was still upset about their earlier request to learn balance and was allowing that to cloud her perception. They informed Ellen that everything was quite alright and then left her again, to her own devices. What a terrible day for our elephant. Later that night, there was a tiny knock at the bottom of the entrance to her room. Ellen told the knocker to come in, half out of habit. The tiny brown mouse stood to wait in the doorway.

"I am so sorry that I gave you such a fright earlier. It was wrong of me to be in your room without permission. I was looking for straw for my own house. I really did not mean to frighten you. My name is Ida." The mouse said.

"Take anything you want, except for my bow!" Ellen screamed back. She was visibly shaken by the mouse's presence, and willing to do anything to rid herself of this tiny monster.

"Tell me Elephant, why are you so terrified of me?" The mouse asked.

Ellen explained that she was compulsively worried that something as tiny as this crafty little mouse might run right up her trunk. This seemed to be a fear that all elephants possessed, and she was surely not alone in this belief. Ida shook her head in dismay, knowing that there is no way that this elephant has ever had an experience even remotely like the one

282

that she has been envisioning. This sort of thinking led to a lot of negative mouse stereotypes. Even if Ida had a habit of breaking into rooms and stealing trash, she'd never even think of clogging up someone else's nose tube thing (mice aren't hyperaware of elephant body parts). She did her best to explain to the elephant that she was actually a huge fan of her performance and had often wondered what it would be like to be on stage herself. Ellen found herself feeling more and more comfortable with the mouse as their conversation went on. She even confided in Ida about the trainers and their request that she overcomes her natural clumsiness. Ellen then talked at length about how she knew that she could never be as graceful as some of the other animals. Ida had always been a good listener. She took the time to really understand Ellen's hesitation with the request, before finally offering her advice:

"Please don't think of it as the trainers asking you to change a part of your personality. They're asking you to evolve into a better performer. You aren't going to be a baby forever, and someday you will need to know how to get around without hurting yourself. Becoming better is never a bad thing and if you think that you can't do it… well, you are just wrong. You need to change your thought process around change; change is a wonderful thing. Change is how you become the person that you're meant to be. Instead of tearing yourself down, you should build yourself up. Practice your heart and know that you can overcome this obstacle just like every obstacle." The mouse said.

Ellen was quiet for a moment while she considered Ida's words. She hadn't even considered that they were preparing her for the future. She thought that the trainers wanted her to change as an attack on her talent as a performer. She agreed to try her best to become more graceful and she asked her new friend to help her train. The next day the two set out to teach Ellen balance and awareness of her surroundings. Ida sat atop her head and pointed out every unlevel piece of ground as they traversed a field behind the circus. Ellen was unsteady on the first day of practice and became more and more frustrated as the day went on. She stumbled over her ears swayed from one side to the other. Ellen sighed and sat on the edge of the field, upset with herself for failing. Ida, still clinging to the top of the small elephant's head, was having none of this. She explained that failure is a necessary step in the process of mastering a skill.

"My first house was a wreck, easily found and destroyed by larger animals. The next time I built a house, I did so in a more secluded environment. Every time I rebuild, my houses get better and better. This does not defeat; it's only your first step in the process." The mouse explained.

The next day, the pair returned to the field. They tied Ellen's ears back with her favorite bow and there was an instant change. The little elephant was able to see all around herself now and no longer had to worry about tripping over every rock they crossed. Ida realized that this whole time, her ears had been the issue. The two of them still practiced all day, but the difference in Ellen's stride was remarkable. From that week on, the two were inseparable. Ida rebuilt her house in Ellen's room and two stayed up laughing late into the night, every night. If Ellen had let her fear get the better of her, to this day she would be a clumsy elephant with no best friend.

Soon Ellen had convinced the trainers to let Ida try out for the circus too. She was such a talented little mouse, that the circus was eager to have her. Ida and Ellen became known worldwide as The Unlikely Duo, and eventually, they performed all of their acts together. Ellen insisted that Ida take one of her favorite pink bows to that they could match on stage. Ida was especially nimble and excellent at acrobatic tricks, though ensuring that the audience could see her was not always the simplest task. One of the more industrious trainers actually invented a huge magnifying glass that became a staple in their acts. The trainers would roll out the enormous contraption and the crowd would go wild. Watching in eager anticipation as the mouse flipped around Ellen, who was always very careful to gently catch Ida with her trunk.

Then Ellen would dance around the ring as though rhythm and grace were gifts, she was given at birth. She would sashay around throwing out one foot at a time. The audience loved her, and her best friend Ida and they continued to be a favorite attraction for many years to come. The most treasured of their shows involved Ida pretending to scare Ellen, who would then run through a very difficult obstacle course that consisted of many challenging jumps and twists. In a playful spirit, they named this act The Mouse of Doom.

CHAPTER 22

Pame's Ordeal

A fter many years of waiting, Mr. &Mrs. Ontai was blessed with a male child. The baby was indeed a miracle because he came at a time when all hope was lost. On the day of the naming, people came from far and near to rejoice with them. The naming ceremony was a big one because there was enough to eat, drink and even take away. So many people blessed the couple and the newborn baby many gifts. He was christened, Pame.

As a child born after so many years of barrenness and also, being a couple who were rich, the mother over-pampered the child right from when he was still suckling. The mother could not stand seeing her baby cry for any reason. Immediately she gave birth, she hired four caregivers who took a turn to sleep in the same room with the baby. They ran shift; two per day, one will be there during the day, another one will sleep there at night. At night, once the baby makes a sound, the nurse must wake up to quickly go and call the mother to breastfeed Pame. Peradventure, the baby cries and the mother hears before the nurse gets to her, she gets fired immediately. Pame lacked nothing. He grew like every other child but swam in so much luxury that he lacked nothing. Mr. Ontai never liked the way the mother was handling Pame but the mother wouldn't listen. Whenever he raises the issue, the mother will say she wants the best for her child and she is going to do everything in her capacity to make sure she gave her child the best.

The first-day Pame was to start school was a challenging one for the mother as she has never allowed him out of her sight. She made sure the nurse followed her to school every day with the driver who drives them. Everyone in the neighborhood saw how the mother treated her only son like an egg. In school, no teacher is permitted to rebuke him no matter what his offense might be. Any teacher who does that will see the full wrath of his mother. If he got in a fight with someone, the mother was always supporting her son even if she knows that her son is wrong. This made so many people dislike Pame including his nurses and even his classmates. They saw him as a spoilt brat.

He also grew up to become so proud. He wanted everything to be in his favor. Anytime he reports any of his nurses, such will be fired immediately and so, the nurses always entreated his favor. One day, Pame was in the sitting room watching TV, one of the nurses was also clearing the dining table after eating. All of a sudden, he picked up the flower vase on the center table and broke it. Unknown to him, his father was watching him from a distance. When the mother heard the sound, she ran to the sitting room and asked what happened, Pame said, "Miss Jeanne broke the flower vase. She picked it and broke it". All the nurse's explanation fell on Mrs. Ontai's deaf ears as she kept saying, "how can you break the precious flower vase that cost me a fortune to buy". The lady kept pleading that she knew nothing about it but the woman wouldn't have it. After some minutes, the father came around and the following conversation ensued.

Mr. Ontai: Pame, are you sure it was Miss Jeanne who broke the vase

Pame nodded in the affirmative while he answered with his mouth and said, "yes".He probed further, "where were you seated when the flower vase broke?"

Pame squeezed his face and said, "I was sitting right here in the sitting room watching my favorite TV program".

While all these were going on, Mrs. Ontai, on the other hand, was uncomfortable with the questions because she felt asking questions had nothing to do with the fact that it was the nurse who broke her vase. She just stood there fuming with anger while the nurse kept pleading her innocence. Unmoved by what his wife was doing, he asked the nurse, " where were you when you heard the sound?". The nurse answered amidst tears, "I had just finished eating and was packing plates to the kitchen to go and wash when I heard the sound sir". Mr. Ontai finally spoke up and said, "I saw everything that happened, it wasn't the nurse that broke the vase". Immediately he said that his wife flared up and said, "then, who broke my vase? I am so sure it can't be my dear son". Mr. Ontai replied to her and said, " it was your son who broke your vase. I was watching from a distance and I saw everything that happened. He took it deliberately and smashed it on the floor thinking nobody was looking". The moment he said that the boy bowed his head in shame while the mother was trying to defend her son. She said, "it must be a mistake then. Maybe he was playing with it". The man shook his head and asked the nurse to wipe her face and get to work. He then turned to his wife and said, "I pray you don't regret all of these". She just hissed and said, "I will do everything to protect the interest of my only son". She walked out of the man holding her little boy. These and many more made this boy develop a thick skin and he no longer felt any remorse for any wrongdoing. He was full of lies.

The boy, Pame grew worse as he grew older. To make matters worse, he was a dullard. He found it difficult to retain anything he is being taught. He doesn't read and he wasn't willing to learn. Of course, he had friends who were like him. They were also from rich families and they were also spoilt brats. They always disturb the class whenever any teaching was going on. They were bullies, they bullied their classmates and people who were older than them. Yet, in all of these, the mother kept encouraging him in all of his deeds while his father made up his mind never to be a part of the evil.

Years passed and he made it out of college with just a pass that couldn't even get him a job. He continued with his friendship with those boys and they were always partying. A time came that they felt they were

288

big boys and the money their parents were giving wasn't enough to sustain them and can't also secure a job. Then, they resorted to pickpocketing. They will steal money from people without the victims being aware. Mr. & Mrs. Ontai had grown older and the reality of everything began to dawn on Mrs. Ontai but she couldn't undo the past. She was full of regret while the father, on the other hand, wasn't happy with the way Pame was living.

On a fateful day, Pame and the boys went to a shopping mall to carry out their evil plans as usual. They divided themselves into different sections and they were picking monies from unsuspecting victims. Unknown to them, there was a CCTV camera that was capturing what was going on and information had been sent to the security personnel at the entrance. So, the security personnel started carrying out a stop-and-search operation on everyone. As they were about to leave, they were also searched and they discovered some monies on them and because the security personnel had their pictures, they arrested them and whisked them away.Information got to their parents that their children had been arrested. Immediately, Mrs. Ontai heard of the news, she fainted and was rushed to the hospital. The father was devastated as he was shuttling between the hospital and the cell. They were charged to court and Pame's father hired a good lawyer just to make sure that Pame wasn't sentenced to prison. The judge finally gave his verdict and sentenced all of them to ten years imprisonment with hard labor. All of them were handcuffed and were led away. The mother was watching the court proceeding from the hospital and immediately she heard the news, she gave up the ghost. Mr. Ontai too passed away a few years as he couldn't bear the pain.

CHAPTER 23

David Goes Whale Watching

H ave you ever wondered what it would be like to head out to the sea and go whale watching with your family?

Whale watching is a wonderful experience that is enjoyed by many who live near the beautiful ocean.

In tonight's story, we are going to talk about how David went whale watching with his family and all of the wonderful experiences he had and the emotions he learned about as he went.

Before we start our story, make sure that you are ready for bed!

Say goodnight to your family, brush your teeth, and get a drink of water.

If you have a favorite blanket or stuffed animal, you like to sleep with, snuggle up close with them and get ready for a wonderful night's sleep.

Then, when you are ready, we can spend a few minutes breathing to help you relax with a calming meditation before we start tonight's story.

That way, your body is nice and relaxed and ready to stay still while you listen to the story and prepare yourself for a wonderful dream.

For this breathing meditation, we are going to breathe in for the count of five, hold it for two seconds, and breathe out to the count of seven.

This helps you relax your mind, and it tells your body that it is time to calm down and go to sleep.

Now, let your breath go back to normal as you settle in for a wonderful story about David and his whale watching experience.

David was so excited to go visit his family on the coast.

He spent the whole week packing his bags.

He packed his pants, his shirts, his underwear, his socks, his shoes, and even a few of his favorite toys.

In a smaller bag, he packed his toothbrush, toothpaste, shampoo, conditioner, and a small towel.

All of his bags were ready to go on Friday morning when it was time for him and his parents to make the drive to the coast where they would stay with David's grandparents for the weekend.

David was so excited to see his grandparents as he had not seen them in months, and he missed them dearly.

The whole way there, he excitedly talked about what they would do, how they would spend their time, and what fun it would be to spend this weekend with his grandparents.

To help him contain his excitement, his parents encouraged him to play games like counting how many telephone poles he saw in one town, or counting how many green cars he saw along the way.

David played along and counted out 19 telephone poles, and 37 green cars.

After what seemed like forever, David and his parents arrived at the coast and at his grandparent's house.

His grandparents were just as excited to see him as he was to see them, and they enjoyed a wonderful evening eating his grandma's delicious spaghetti and meatballs with a slice of cake for dessert.

That night, he slept in the guest room with a big smile on his face because he was so excited to be with his grandparents again.

When the next morning came, David woke up and saw that his grandparents and his parents were packing some bags.

"Are we leaving already?" David frowned.

"No, not at all. We are going on an adventure today!" David's grandpa exclaimed.

"An adventure? Where?" David asked.

"It's a surprise." his grandpa grinned.

"Before the adventure, you need a good breakfast to help you get started with your day!

Come on, let's enjoy some pancakes and bacon before we leave." David's grandma said, calling everyone into the dining room.

Everyone went and ate their breakfasts, and it was delicious.

When they were done, they cleaned their plates.

"Is it time for the adventure now?" David asked.

"It sure is!" his grandpa grinned, giving him a thumbs up.

David, his parents, and his grandparents all got their shoes on and got ready to leave the house.

While they were on their way to the adventure, David felt excited and confused.

He had no idea what they were getting up to, but he knew it was going to be a good time because he always had fun with his grandparents.

As they drove, David started to see the ocean in front of them.

He could see it getting bigger and bigger as they drove closer.

"Are we going to the beach?" he asked.

"Sort of." his mom said, keeping their adventure a mystery.

David grew even more curious as they drove closer and closer to the beach, and eventually parked in a parking lot near the water.

292

"We are going to the beach, aren't we?" he said, excited.

"You'll see." his dad grinned.

His parents and grandparents picked up some of the bags out of the trunk and locked the car as they began walking toward a small building on the beach.

When they got there, David saw tons of pictures and statues of whales on the building.

"What are we doing, grandpa?" he asked, looking around in wonder.

"We're going whale watching!" his grandpa responded.

"Whale watching? I have never been! This is so exciting!" David said, jumping all around.

His parents and grandparents smiled as they checked in, and everyone got ready to go whale watching.

When they were all checked in, one of the guides leads David and his family to the boat that they would use to go whale watching.

Each of them climbed aboard and found a seat to sit on as they relaxed and watched out toward the sea.

David was so excited about what was going on that he could hardly contain himself, but the whale watching guide told him it was important that he sit down and stay still so that he does not accidentally hurt himself or fall off the boat.

Then, the guide handed each of them life jackets and told them what to do if they did fall out of the boat or if anything happened.

He assured them that it was unlikely that anyone would fall out, but that it was important that he tell them what to do anyway just in case.

As David listened to the guide, he looked over the edge of the boat and realized how far away the water was.

293

He started to grow scared as he realized what might happen if he moved, so he sat incredibly still.

In fact, he sat so still that David's grandma wondered if something was wrong.

"Are you okay?" she asked.

"I am, I am just scared of falling into the water. I have never fallen into the ocean before, what if I get hurt?" he asked.

"You will be okay, just stay relaxed and close to grandpa and I and we will keep you safe." David's dad assured him.

He was sitting between his dad and grandpa, and, realizing that he was not alone, he started to feel more comfortable.

For the first little while out on the water, David felt scared.

He worried that something might happen and that they would get hurt.

Once they had been out for a while, though, David began to settle down.

He relaxed so much that he was able to laugh at the jokes that his grandpa was telling as they enjoyed the view and a wonderful time together.

Soon, they made it to the point where the whales were, and the guide told them to look up.

David looked out where the guide was pointing and saw the backs of whales as they bobbed through the water.

They seemed to be playing and dancing in the waves as they swam around.

One even sprayed water up into the air higher than their boat!

The guide carefully moved the boat a little closer so that they could get a better view.

David was surprised by how beautiful and fascinating the whales were to watch.

When he asked to go closer, the guide told him they had to stay further away so that the whales did not get hurt.

The guide said that sometimes the whales became so curious about the boats they would come to touch them with their noses, and they might get hurt by the propellers.

David did not want the whales to get hurt so he agreed they should keep their distance and enjoy the whales from afar.

They sat there for a while and watched the whales dancing in the waves as they enjoyed the sunlight.

It seemed as though they were all playing together, and David thought that was cute.

After a while, the whales began to disappear.

The other boats that had also been whale watching began to head back toward shore, and their guide suggested that David's family start going back toward shore, too.

"Aw, but I don't want to! I'm having fun!" David said.

"I know, but we have to say goodbye to the pod of whales and let them have a good sleep!" David's mom said.

"What is a pod of whales?"

"A pod is what you call a group of whales." his mom answered.

"Oh. Bye pod of whales!" David said, waving at the whales.

The guide began to take David and his family back to shore.

When they got there, they took their life jackets off and one by one they got off the boat.

His parents went to talk to the guide while David and his grandparents brought their bags back to the car.

When his parents were done talking, they all got back into the car and started to head back to his grandparent's house.

Slowly, the ocean grew further and further away as they went back toward the suburbs where his grandparents lived.

Before he knew it, they were back home and ready to enjoy a wonderful dinner together.

David was tired, but he stayed awake long enough to enjoy dinner with his grandparents and his family.

When dinner was ready, they all sat down together at the table and enjoyed a wonderful meal.

They had ham, mashed potatoes, carrots, gravy, corn, and buns.

When that was done, David and his family enjoyed another slice of his favorite cake for dessert, and David even got to have a few of the cookies his grandma often ate with her tea after dinner.

As they were sitting down enjoying the evening, his grandma asked: "David, what was your favorite part of today?"

"My favorite part was seeing the pod of whales playing in the waves. It looked like they were dancing! And when the whale sprayed water into the air!" David said, making a grand gesture into the air as if he were the whale spraying water.

David's parents and grandparents giggled as they watched him act out the part of the whales.

When he was done, David sat down on the couch and began to fall asleep.

"Are you tired?" his mom asked.

"Yes," David whispered.

David's dad carried him to the guest room where he was tucked in so that he could enjoy a wonderful night's sleep after a great day of whale watching with his family. The end!

Going on adventures can be fun, but they can also sometimes be scary.

When you do not know what you are doing, it can be scary to try new things.

The good thing is, you do not have to go on adventures alone, and you can always rely on your loved ones to help you feel safe.

When you know that you are going to be safe while going on an adventure, adventures can be great fun and can lead to wonderful lifelong memories.

You may not realize it now, but these memories will be very special to you!

As you test out new adventures in your own life, I encourage you to keep these affirmations close by to help you feel confident when taking adventures:

"It is safe to go on adventures."

"Adventures with my family are fun."

"Trying new things is great."

"I feel my feelings when I try new things."

"Adventure is fun."

"I love adventures with my family."

"I listen to the rules when I go on adventures."

"Listening to the rules helps me stay safe."

"Adventures can be a great time."

"These memories will last forever."

CHAPTER 24

The Greedy Tortoise

Mr. Tortoise was someone given to greed. He loved the food so much that no one dared compete with him. All his neighbors knew him as a glutton. If Tortoise makes friends today, it will be because of food and if he stops being a friend with someone, it's still because of food.

Once, he was a friend to Mr. Turtle who loved him so much. They spend most of their time together. Everyone in the community knew them as friends. So many times, Tortoise ate from Turtle because he knows Tortoise is not too rich and can't afford his meals. Though Turtle was selfless in everything he did for Tortoise but Tortoise on the other hand never really loved Turtle. He was just moving with him because of the food he usually gets from him. At a time, Turtle needed to go and visit his sick parents in the next village and he didn't want to take his two children with him. He began to think of what to do and then, he remembered he had a friend, Tortoise. Without delay, he went to Tortoise's house and explained to him that he needs to visit his parents and that he is going to spend some time and he wants his children to stay with Tortoise. Mr. Tortoise quickly responded, "You are my good friend. Whatever you have is mine and vice versa. Be rest assured that I will take care of your children". The turtle was happy and thanked him. Well, Tortoise was happy because that was an opportunity for him to enjoy himself.

When Turtle was leaving, he took his two children to Tortoise's house and went with plenty of food for the children and Tortoise, he was not yet married at the time. When he left, Tortoise gave them enough food for about two days and began to starve them. Sometimes, he gave them a small portion of food for breakfast and will not give them lunch but give them a small portion for dinner while he ate more than enough for breakfast, lunch and dinner. He gave them food whenever he liked and the children couldn't do anything. The children began to grow lean because they were starved. Before Turtle came back, the food had finished.

After some time, the Turtle came back and was happy to see his children and his friend. Though, he noticed his children were lean, yet, he thanked his friend for taking care of them in his absence. When they got home, he never allowed his children to report his friend to him. Even though he noticed he didn't take care of his children as he would have loved, he never allowed it to affect their friendship. He continued being good to him.

Both of them had a friend, Mr. Crocodile whom they visit once a while. One day, Tortoise decided to go and greet Crocodile before going to Turtle's place. When he got to his place, they greeted each other as it had been long, they saw. Crocodile offered him a seat and they began to gist. The crocodile then asked of their third friend, Turtle and he said, "Oh, Turtle is fine. He just got back from his parent's place". Crocodile replied, "That's good". Tortoise continued, "He even put his children in my place. He made me a nanny and well, it was an opportunity to enjoy myself as I feasted well on his food". Unknown to him, Turtle was also outside and had come to greet Crocodile and was about entering when he heard what he said. He then entered and greeted both of them and told Tortoise right there never to visit his place again. Tortoise begged Turtle but he wouldn't accept his plea. Crocodile also joined in begging but he didn't agree. That was how their friendship ended.

Tortoise began to plan on how to make new friends so that he can get food to eat as he doesn't joke with food. He started moving close to Ms. Hawk. He started getting nice towards her. Whenever she needed help, he was always there to help. He was doing all of

300

those to entreat her favor. At first, Hawk didn't trust him because she knows he can be very cunning but when he told her that he had changed, she believed him.

While he was at her place one day, one of the birds came and told Hawk that there is going to be a get together for all birds in the sky and that there would be more than enough to eat and drink, his body was already shaking and planning on how to be there. When the bird left, Tortoise told Hawk that she would love to follow the birds but she refused him saying he was not a bird and doesn't have wings. The tortoise then told her that if she loves him as a friend, she will arrange how she will get there. After much persuasion, she told him she will try her best. She then spoke to other birds to please borrow Tortoise one feather each so that he can fly with them and that when he comes back, he will return the feathers.

The birds agreed to borrow him. On the day of the event, they all met at Hawk's house and each of them gave a feather to Tortoise and even helped him attach the feathers to his body and when they finished, they all flew to the event. When they got to the party, they were well entertained. Tortoise told all of them that he would like to be the one to go and carry food and even serve them because they did him a favor. Unknown to them, he had a plan. When he had collected the food and meats, he went to a corner and shared the food into two halves, then, kept one part and took the other half to them. The birds were surprised at the small quantity of food but they didn't suspect any foul play. He shared the food and meat and they all ate.

When they finished eating, he excused himself to use the toilet and off, he went to the portion he kept and began to eat. Parrot decided to go and urinate and when he was passing, he saw Tortoise at one corner eating. That was when she knew what Tortoise did. She went to the other birds and told them what she saw. All of them followed her and met him where he was eating. He was so ashamed of himself and couldn't say anything. Out of anger, they all asked him to give them back

301

their feathers. Though he begged they wouldn't listen. They all removed their leather and he was left with nothing.

He then asked them for a favor but none answered but later, Bat decided to help him. He then told Bat to help him tell his neighbor to help him bring out his bed and chairs so that when he jumps from the sky, he will land on them. When Bat got to his house, he told Tortoise's neighbor that he asked him to bring out the cutlasses, hoes, and knives he had at home. That one did as he was told. When Tortoise jumped from the sky, he landed on the sharp objects and his shell scattered on the floor. He was badly injured. He had to get someone to help him put the shell together but it was never smooth again. That was how his shell became rough since then.

CHAPTER 25

Tommy Gets a New Friend

Tommy was an ace in the water. He had been swimming and snorkeling since he was a toddler. His Dad took him down to the sea when he was a newborn, and held him in his arms while he walked up and down the beach talking to his new son. Something had happened in those early times that Tommy could not quite grasp, but he knew one thing for sure. He loved the ocean; he loved everything about it. The white sands, the blue water, and what could be out there in the deeps? He did not know, but he was going to find out, and now he had a much better understanding of how that would take shape. Dragons!

Tommy had brought his snorkeling gear and was sitting up against the rocks, getting ready to go into the water, when he heard a sound in his head. "Hello, Tommy!" It was baby Drake, and Tommy was thrilled. Meeting Drake was the first meaningful psychic conversation he had experienced, and he was excited to learn more about his powers and the strange new creature who had come up from the depths to apparently meet him, or so he thought.

"Is that you, Drake? Where are you?" Tommy mentally asked. "Still full of questions, I see." Drake replied and, "I am out at the end of the point. Is anyone there around you, or on the beach near where you are?" Drake asked. Tommy looked around but saw no one. "I am here at the point, and I do not see anyone," Tommy informed Drake. "Okay, then I'm coming in." was all that the little dragon said. It wasn't long before Tommy saw him again. He came up out of the water very near to where

Tommy was sitting and walked across the sand to sit beside his new friend.

"You may ask any questions you have now," the dragon said. "Thank you," Tommy said and began to think of what to ask and how to word the questions so as not to make the testy little guy angry again. He began. "Do you have parents, and where do you live?" Tommy asked. "Yes, and we live not far from here on the bottom, in a large cave that is filled with air. The cave is a very old and sacred place that we dragons have been visiting for centuries, and my Mother and Father live there, as well as my two older sisters. Would you like to meet them?" Drake asked. All this was nearly too much for little Tommy, so he thought for a moment and then gathered his wits and began to speak. "I would be honored to meet your family if they would have me." Was all he said. "Good, very good, my friend," said the little dragon.

They talked for a good hour before both going into the water to swim. Tommy swam down into the shallows of the lagoon, and Drake was there right beside him. Drake found interesting things, and Tommy picked them up, and they went back up and onto the beach to check out their artifacts. This they did for the next three hours, and Tommy found his new friend to be a great company. They found some old plates, and an old rusty lantern, and something else that was mostly buried that they could not pull out of the sea bottom. Tommy told Drake that he would bring something to dig with tomorrow, and they said goodbye for the day, and Tommy headed home.

That night, Tommy awakened suddenly to voices in his head. He could not determine what it was or why he was hearing them, and eventually, he fell back asleep. In the morning, like all mornings, breakfast with his Mom and Dad, and then back to the beach, only this time, he brought a small camping shovel.

Much to his surprise, there was Drake, sitting upon a rock sunning himself.

304

"Good morning Tommy," Drake said. "Hi there, Mr. Dragon," Tommy responded.

"Did you hear us talking last night?" Drake asked. "Yes, I did. So that was you, after all. I wondered about that." Tommy said, mentally to Drake. "Why did I hear you, but you were not talking directly to me?" Tommy asked. "Oh that," Drake said, looking down at the rocks. "Well, actually, I'm new at this psychic stuff, and I was talking to my parents, and it just sorts of slipped out. I kinda turned it on by mistake, so you really were not supposed to hear any of that, but no matter."

Drake replied. "You know, I was worried about the very same thing," Tommy said to Drake. "I guess there is no rule book for this psychic communication stuff is there?" Tommy stated, and "Well, I know one thing for sure, and that is, if I am mindful, my thoughts should be just my own. What I mean to say is that nobody else should be able to hear my thoughts, right?" Tommy said.

"Drake," Tommy suddenly said, "I want to talk to you about something. You are a tiny dragon, and I am a tiny human, so I guess we are both kinds of in the same boat if you know what I mean. What I want to say is that my parents have always taken me to church on Sunday mornings. Always! I mean, we never miss church. I think it has always meant a lot to them, but anyhow this church is not exactly like a normal church. I mean, we pray and read the Bible and sing hymns, but there is much more to it. They have classes that my parents have always made me go to after each service that teach something sort of different than other churches do. It is called mindful meditation. Have you ever heard of that?" Tommy asked the dreary eyed little dragon. "Wow, that was a mouthful you just said. No, I can't say I've ever heard of mindful meditation, but we practice fire breathing. Is it anything like that?" Drake asked.

Tommy burst out laughing and thought the little Dragon was only kidding. Drake's eyes became really huge, and he made a sort of gurgling growling sound deep down in his throat. "Uh, Oh, did I make you

305

mad?" Tommy asked. "Well, it sounded like you thought that a very big part of my life was funny!" Drake snarled. "Oh, no-no-no," Tommy quickly snapped. "Really, I just thought you were…. Uh, well, I guess I wasn't listening right, that must be it. So, tell me more about this fire breathing thing you do then." Tommy gasped. He didn't want to lose his only friend, and certainly didn't want to be on the receiving end of a burst of flames!

"Well, we dragons by nature have certain abilities, and that is one of them. I guess you could say it would be a little bit like our ability to use mental communication. I think the off worldly call that telepathy." A more calm Drake stated. Just then, a group of tourists could be seen clambering up the jetty from the other side. Since Drake had his back to the jetty, he didn't see them. "Quick, back in the water. Somebody is coming!" Tommy gasped, whereby the little dragon dove headlong into the shallows near the jetty. As the tourists appeared in full force upon the jetty, Tommy waved hello to them, hoping they had not caught sight of the dragon.

The situation returned to normal, the tourists faded out of sight down the beach, and Drake's head bobbed up some distance out in the water. Tommy just beckoned to him and then noticed the dragon moving closer to him. "That was close." The dragon said, and "I don't like being spotted by strangers, as you may recall from the odd meeting on the fishing boat." Tommy chuckled and said, "I think that was planned actually, don't you?" he asked. "Okay my friend, I guess you already know that we wanted to make contact with you, is that what you are thinking then?" Drake asked. "Well, I am just glad you did because you know I have these abilities, these powers, and I'm just a kid of 9, so I'm still sorting everything out myself," Tommy explained.

The two chatted for another hour, and then agreed to meet again the next day; same time, same place. "Good, Okay then see you tomorrow Drake," Tommy said, and with that, the little dragon again dove into the shallows and was gone. Tommy sat there thinking for a good deal of time after Drake left. He was putting together a plan in his mind as to how to learn more about all this. He would have to run it by the dragon tomorrow. With that, Tommy picked up his things and rode home.

The evening was mundane, and Tommy went to bed, but he could not stop thinking about Drake. He thought that just maybe he would "call" Drake up with his mind and say goodnight. Yes, he thought, that would be an experiment for me so I can figure this telepathy thing out. Tommy used his mindfulness and cleared his thoughts. Then, he did some meditation and used his third eye technique to calm himself even further. After that, in his mind, he said, "Drake, can you hear me?" Boom! Just like magic, Drake was there in his mind. "Hi Tommy, how are you?" Drake said. "Just wanted to reach out and say thanks for meeting me today." Tommy thought. "Sure, no problem, it was fun. We'll talk again tomorrow. Good night." The dragon said, and "Good night, my friend, until tomorrow then." And with that, Tommy signed off. That was easy, Tommy thought. "I guess it's just all about mindfulness and meditation, isn't it?" Tommy thought to himself and then fell into a deep sleep.

CHAPTER 26

Noah Rides an Airplane

There are many ways to travel where you want to go. Trains, cars, trucks, buses, and boats are all great modes of transportation. Another great mode of transportation is airplanes. Airplanes fly high in the sky above everything, helping people get to their special destination with ease. For many people, airplanes are a mode of transportation that they use on a regular basis to help them get where they are going. For example, politicians and musicians use airplanes to get to important meetings or concerts that they are hosting all over the world! For Noah, airplanes were brand new. He had never been on an airplane before, and he had no idea what to expect. But, Noah's grandpa wanted to take him on a special trip to the other side of the country to visit a special museum, but he could only do that if they were going to fly. Trying to drive that far would take a very long time, and trains were more expensive to ride on and often took longer to get to their destinations. With an airplane, though, Noah and his grandpa would be across the country in just a couple of hours. Noah thought it was very cool that a plane could travel so fast, and that they would get there in almost no time at all. As they were getting ready for their trip, Noah began to get nervous. He was excited to ride in an airplane with his grandpa, but the idea of going somewhere new and then being so high scared Noah. He did not know what it would be like to go through the airport or to ride in an airplane. Noah worried that maybe he would get scared, or that he would feel uncomfortable while he and his grandpa rode the airplane.

While he packed his bags and got ready for his trip, Noah's dad tried to comfort him so that Noah would feel more comfortable with the trip he was going to take with his grandpa.

Noah's dad told Noah that taking the airplane would be easy. He told him that they would check in their luggage, and the airport attendees would make sure their luggage got on their airplane. Then, they would be checked through security to make sure they were not carrying anything that might be unsafe to carry on an airplane. Next, they would wait in a big sitting area for their airplane to be called; then, they would get on the airplane. Once they were on, they would fasten their seatbelts and listen to the pilot tell them what to expect. Then, they could watch TV on the airplane while a flight attendant brought them snacks and drinks. Noah's dad told him that by the time they were done eating and drinking, the flight would almost be done, and they would get off. Then, they would get their luggage from the luggage trolley and make their way to their car so that they could go to the museum! Noah did not think that it sounded too hard to ride an airplane, but still, he was worried about all of these new experiences. That night, he had a difficult time sleeping as he wondered what it was going to be like and how he would do during his first time flying. Even though Noah was scared, he was still very excited to go on this special adventure with his grandpa.

The next morning, it was time for Noah's ride on an airplane. His grandpa came to his house and put his bags in the car while Noah said goodbye to his parents. By now, he was feeling both very scared and very excited about this special trip he was taking with his grandpa. After he was done saying goodbye to his parents, Noah and his grandpa got in the car and headed toward the airport. Noah told his grandpa that he was scared and excited at the same time, and Noah's grandpa said he understood. Then, he told Noah the same things his dad had told him about what to expect and how easy it would be to take the flight. Noah started to feel more comfortable and tried to relax as they made their way to the airport.

309

When they got to the airport, Noah's grandpa parked their car in a special parking lot, and then they paid for a special ticket that let Noah's grandpa leave his car there until they got home. This way, they would have a car to drive home in when they got back from their trip! Once the fare was paid, they walked into the airport and started the process of getting ready to get on the plane. First, they went to the luggage area and gave their bags to the luggage attendants. As they did, the luggage attendants placed tags on their bags that let the airport know which flight those bags needed to be on. Then, they signed papers to confirm that their bags had been checked and kept a piece of paper for confirmation. Once they checked their bags in, they made their way to the security checkpoint. This part felt scary for Noah, as there were many sounds, machines, and people all over the place. Everyone had formed lines toward the checkpoint so that the security guards could make sure that everyone was safe and ready to travel.

This part took a while as it took time for each person to be checked in through the checkpoint in order for them to get to the waiting room. Noah watched as each person took off their jackets, shoes, and any jewelry that they might be wearing to put them in a bucket with their bags. The bucket would then go down a conveyer belt through a metal detector, and then the people would walk through a separate metal detector. On the other side, the security guard would make sure everything looked proper and safe, and then they would let the passenger through to the waiting area. Finally, it was Noah and his grandpa's turn to go through the security pass. Each of them took off their shoes and their jackets, and Noah's grandpa took off his wristwatch. Then, they put their carryon bags on the conveyer belt. One by one, they walked through the metal detector, and their bags went through the metal detector, too.

On the other side, the security guard checked to make sure that everything was okay, and then they were given their stuff back. They put their shoes and jackets back on, and Noah's grandpa put his wristwatch back on. Then, they grabbed their carryon bags and headed to the

310

waiting area. The waiting area was just a big lounge filled with chairs and a few airport stores. One store was a convenience store with snacks and drinks, and the other was a book store. There was also a restaurant in case people wanted to eat before they took their flight to wherever they were going. Noah looked around at all of the people who were waiting, eating, and shopping for books. He was surprised by how many people were in the waiting area and wondered how many of them would be taking the flight with him and his grandpa. Noah and his grandpa found a seat and waited for the attendant to call their number so that they could board their airplane. When she did, they got up and went to the lineup, showed the attendant their boarding pass, and then started to board. Boarding the airplane was unusual: they walked down a long hallway and ended up on the plane at the end. Noah thought it was cool that they could attach this hallway to the airplane and that they could get on the airplane this way. Once they were on the airplane, Noah and his grandpa found their seats and sat down. It took a while for everyone to board the airplane.

Noah and his grandpa watched as families, men, women, and business folks all piled on. Each one found their seats, put their bags away, and then sat down and waited as the rest of the passengers boarded. Finally, after what seemed like forever, everyone was on board, and the airplane was ready to take off. They started takeoff with a message from the pilot.

The pilot talked to them about the flying conditions, and what to expect in terms of turbulence. Then, he talked to them about safety measures and what to do if there was a problem with the airplane.

This made Noah worry, but his grandpa assured him that everything would be fine. When the pilot was done talking, the big TV at the front of the plane turned on, and Noah was offered headphones from the flight attendant. He and his grandpa each accepted a pair and turned them on so that they could listen to the movie that was being played while they flew.

Then, they took off.

Take off was a cool experience for Noah. It started with them driving down the runway, but soon they were going so fast that the plane took off into the air. They took a sharp turn upward, and within moments they were flying through the clouds. Soon, they were above the clouds and flying straight to the other side of the country. Noah looked out the window to see the tops of the clouds and, when the clouds parted, the cities that fell below them. Most of the cities were too far away for Noah to see anything other than the texture of the ground, but he still thought it was very cool. While they flew, Noah looked out the window, watched the TV, and ate the snacks, and drank the drinks that the attendant gave him. Then, just like his dad said, by the time he was done, the plane was almost getting ready to land. As they got closer to their destination, the pilot came on the radio again and told all of the passengers about their landing. He let them know that it was time to put their seatbelts back on and that they would be landing very soon. He told them what time they would be landing at, what to expect, and what to do during the landing process. Soon after, they landed on the runway. It was a bit of a bumpy experience, but it was over quickly. Once they landed, Noah and his grandpa got off the airplane by going down a similar long hallway like the one they had when they boarded the airplane. Then, they went and collected their bags and went outside to catch the taxi to their hotel. The rest of the trip was very exciting for Noah. They stayed in a hotel, went to the museum, and enjoyed delicious dinners and breakfasts from the restaurants near the hotel. By the time their trip was done, Noah was sad to leave all of the fun behind but was excited for another ride on an airplane. Noah thought airplanes were so cool, and he could not wait to go on another trip on an airplane again really soon. He even asked his grandpa if they could go back to the museum again soon! Noah's grandpa just laughed and said sure.

The end!

BEATRICE AND THE WATERMELON

There was once a girl named Beatrice. She was a very lazy girl but finds great pleasure in playing tricks on people and she did not even spare the parents of her naughtiness. She was always failing in school because she never paid attention to her studies.

She had even successfully deceived her mother that she was a seer and has also possessed supernatural abilities to see things that the ordinary eyes cannot see. Her mother, on her part, was extremely happy that her daughter possesses supernatural abilities and she began to tell everyone about the unique powers that she supposedly possessed. The news about Beatrice the seer spread like wildlife and many people came from far and wide to have an experience of her powers.

Beatrice knew how to work her way around the situation hence, she kept on deceiving many people who came to her without them knowing she was deceiving them. She stopped helping her parents in house chores just because she was too powerful to do anything for her parents. She told her parents that they must always respect her as she is more powerful than them. Her parents were not happy with her but there was nothing they could do because she told them that if they got her angry, she could harm them. Both of them decided to leave her.

One day, she went out and came back only to find a businessman waiting for her at home. He had the news that there was a powerful seer in town and he decided to come and visit Beatrice and test her abilities. He said to her, "I need a seer who will help me to make the right decision with his supernatural abilities. I want to buy watermelon fruits and thereafter go and sell it. In this town, so many farmers grow watermelon. I want to know which one sells the sweet one. I promise to build you a house and take you to the city if you can help me but if I lose, I will send you to jail".

Beatrice's eyes shone at the thought of making some quick income. She asked what he wanted her had to do. He told her that he is from a

313

far country and that in his country, the natives love sweet watermelons and so he decided to come to that town to buy watermelon fruits.

She told the man that he should give her some days and that she would get back to him. Right there, she began to plan how to go about her plans so that she will not be caught.

On the second day, she visited the market and did as if she was there to buy fruits. She started moving from one shop to another. When she got to a shop where a woman was selling oranges. She asked for the price and as the woman told her, she began to do as if she was selecting the ones to buy. As she was doing that, she heard the woman and her friend discussing and she started eavesdropping. The owner of the shop told her friend," Mrs. Tim, I heard that the watermelon that just came out is not too sweet and it's just a few people that have the sweet one. I even heard that in this fruit market, only, Mrs. John has the sweet one as today". The other friend was so surprised. She also sells watermelon.

Immediately Beatrice heard, she hurriedly left and went home. She was happy to have successfully done this one too. When she got home, she sent for the businessman and when the man came, she spoke some of her magic languages just for the man to believe she is genuine. She then told the man that the only place he can get the sweet watermelon is from Mrs. John's stall. The man thanked her and told her that he is going to fulfill his promise of building her a house when he is done selling the watermelon fruits. She was so happy that at last, she is going to become a house owner.

Unknown to Beatrice, that very night after she left the market, Mrs. Tim's friend got some people to go Mrs. John's shop to pack all the sweet watermelon fruits and replace them with her own. The following morning, the businessman went to Mrs. John's stall and bought all the woman's watermelon. When he was done buying the watermelon fruits, he went to thank Beatrice and traveled to his town. As he got to his town, he began to tell everyone that he now has the sweetest

314

watermelon in town and everyone should come and buy. People started buying and he was happy.

Before long, people started complaining that the watermelon is not sweet as he said and that he just deceived them. He was so angry and unhappy with their complaints and he decided to have a taste. When he tasted it, it was indeed not sweet. He was so angry that Beatrice deceived him and made him waste his money. He decided to deal with her.

After a week, he went back to the town with police officers who wore mufti. When he got to town, he went straight to Beatrice's house and asked of her. He was told that she wasn't around and he told them he was going to wait for her. When she came back, she was so happy to see the businessman as she was already saying to herself that she is now going to become a house owner. As she exchanged pleasantries with the man, he signaled the officers and they arrested her and thereafter took her away.

Her parents begged the man all to no avail. He told them Beatrice is fake and she is just deceiving people to make herself rich. She was therefore sent to prison. Her parents cried bitterly but there was nothing they could do.

Conclusion

Commentato [WU4]: This has 244 words only. Please add more

I hope that this book has helped you have many wonderful nights' sleep. Let us hope that it was enthralling, as well as thought-provoking and that it provided you with all of the tools you need to get your kids to sleep.

Remember: a good night's sleep is an important part of waking up feeling refreshed and ready to have a great day.

You should always practice doing everything you can to help you have a wonderful night's sleep every single night.

Meditation is not just for sleeping, either!

If you find yourself feeling overwhelmed, angry, stressed out, or even sad, you can always use the important meditation skills you learned right here in this book.

For example, next time you feel overwhelmed, try using the muscle relaxation practice you learned in this book.

Or, the next time you feel angry, try using a helpful breathing meditation.

These skills will help you in many ways in life, so be sure to keep practicing them!

That way, even more kids can have a great sleep!

CPSIA information can be obtained
at www.ICGtesting.com
Printed in the USA
BVHW041141101221
623732BV00013B/481